CANINE ACUPRESSURE

A Treatment Workbook

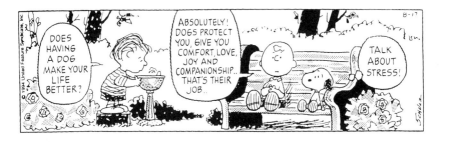

BY:

Nancy A. Zidonis
&
Marie K. Soderberg

Edited By: Mickey Rubin
Cover Art and Illustrations By: Carla Stroh

Published By: Equine Acupressure, Inc.
Printed By: Parker Printing, Inc., Parker, Colorado
Copyright: © 1995 by Equine Acupressure, Inc.

Library of Congress Catalog Number: 95-90259

1st Edition 1995
Printed in the United States of America

ISBN 0-9645982-0-5

To order **Canine Acupressure, A Treatment Workbook,** write to:

> Equine Acupressure Incorporated
> P.O. Box 123
> Parker, Colorado 80134
> 303-841-7211
> Fax 303-841-6939

We are interested in your comments and suggestions regarding the material presented in this book as well as your experience with using acupressure. Please write to us at the above address.

This workbook is not a substitute for veterinary medicine. We suggest that you use acupressure in conjunction with your veterinarian's recommendations.

TABLE OF CONTENTS

1. FOREWORD

This is a workbook for dog owners seeking a way to maintain their dog's health. The treatments and exercises we describe were developed by an acupressurist working in consultation with veterinarians.

We recognize the enormous commitment of time and money many dog owners make to the care of their companions. The acupressure treatments in this book give you, the dog owner, an active role in maintaining and improving your dog's well-being. The treatments use:

1) your relationship with your dog,
2) ancient Oriental medical principles, and
3) a holistic approach to animal well-being.

The treatment program is drug-free and tailored to the needs of the dog. Some programs treat ill or injured dogs. Others are directed at maintaining health or preventing injury. All our treatments are directed at broadening your relationship with your dog while bettering the dog's overall health.

We have worked on both companion dogs and competition dogs. Performance dogs, under the stress of frequent show appearances, have been treated for physical ailments as well as behavioral problems. Our methods successfully remedy soreness, bursitis, lameness, tendinitis, arthritic conditions and behavior problems. We do not claim cures, but we did see significant, lasting improvement in the condition of the dogs we treated—even though conventional techniques had been tried and exhausted.

Acupressure treatment is not limited to a particular breed or age of dog. Our patients have included Golden Retrievers, Boxers, German Short Haired Pointers, Poodles, English Setters, Doberman Pinschers, Great Pyrenees, Basenjis, Cocker Spaniels, German Shepherds, Rottweilers and, of course, several wonderful "mixed" breeds. While acupressure treatments benefit show, performance and working dogs, our methods provide equal benefits to the extraordinary "ordinary" dogs who are our companions and family pets.

We would like to emphasize that this is a workbook, not a comprehensive treatment manual. Acupressure is not a cure-all, but we believe it can help you and your dog. Please remember always to consult your veterinarian in case of an illness or injury to your dog. If you work in partnership with your veterinarian, you will find that acupressure treatments add an important element to your dog's health care, performance routine and quality of life.

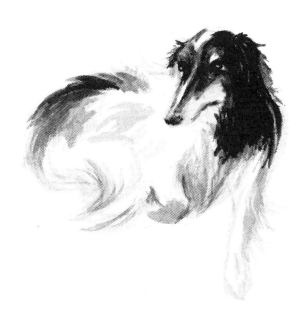

2. INTRODUCTION TO ACUPRESSURE

Before you try acupressure with your dog, you should understand how it differs from more customary treatments. Here is a brief introduction to the history of acupressure, some of its major tenets and the philosophy behind it.

History

Acupressure is an ancient Oriental method of therapy used for a wide variety of human and animal disorders. First developed by the Chinese more than 3,000 years ago, it consists of pressure stimulation of precise points on the surface of the body. This approach to healing differs significantly from western medicine.

According to Western thought, health problems are caused by disease. Conventional medicine, including veterinary science, diagnoses the disease underlying a given complaint and prescribes medication or surgical action to correct the problem.

Oriental medicine, by contrast, is based on the discovery that "points" on the body surface are related to specific internal organs and their functions. By studying different disease states, traditional Oriental medicine has developed a model of the relationships between these surface points, the internal organs and the musculoskeletal system. Stimulating the points can change the functioning of the organs in humans and in animals. Specifically, Chi energy can be dispersed from an area through the technique of "sedation", or Chi can be brought to a deficient area through a technique known as "tonification." With these techniques, points are stimulated in different ways to achieve the desired result, that of restoring a balanced energy flow.

Acupuncture and acupressure both make use of these specific points. Both modalities bring about changes in body energy, the Chinese believe. But while acupuncture involves inserting needles into the body, acupressure does not. Because it is easy to learn and safe to practice, acupressure was used by common people in Japan, China, Korea and Tibet.

Chi Energy

The cornerstone of traditional oriental medicine is the life energy called Chi. In oriental thought, Chi is present in all of nature and is seen in all life forms. Every human and animal is born with a fixed amount of this life energy. Chi flows through the body in pathways known as meridians. The body's meridian system can be looked at as a radio network. The acupressure points are transmitters; the organs act as receivers. The invisible meridian pathways carry messages from the acupressure points to specific parts of the body. Stimulating a point initiates a message.

There are several types of Chi in the human and canine body. These types of Chi are defined by their location and purpose.

- Lung Chi is obtained from the air. It is known by several names including "Chest Chi" or "Big Chi."
- Nutrient Chi is the name given to Chi after the digestive process changes food into body nutrients.
- Source Chi is the hereditary Chi each animal receives at birth.

These three types of Chi are combined throughout the body and course through it by means of the meridian system. As it circulates, the Chi:

- Provides the source of voluntary and involuntary movement;
- Generates body warmth;
- Serves as the basis of organ functions; for example, converting food into nutrients; and
- Protects the body from external harmful forces.

Chi is used in the course of living. Living creatures replenish Chi through food, water, exercise and air. Adding Chi through these sources assures that enough circulates through the body to support healthy functioning. Disease results from an external or internal imbalance in this energy. By stimulating certain points sometimes located far from the site of the symptoms, you can balance vital Chi energy and assist in the healing process.

The Concept of Yin and Yang

Chi energy in its various forms and functions is comprised of the positive and negative forces of yin and yang. These forces are not really distinct, however. They are one. They are most clearly differentiated at the extremes. For example, day is thought of as yang, night as yin. In this example each is clearly defined. However, as day approaches night, or dusk, the distinction between yin and yang becomes less clear. It is here that we can see the reality of one dynamic force.

Despite this, yin and yang are often described as opposites. Some of these attributes are listed below:

Yang	Yin
Excitement	Passivity
Day	Night
Upper	Lower
Hollow	Solid
Hot	Cold
Dry	Moist
Male	Female
Exterior	Interior
Positive	Negative

Chi energy contains both yin and yang aspects. In a healthy body Chi circulates in an on-going balance. In an unhealthy animal, the Chi energy is out of balance. There may be too much or too little yin or yang. The acupressure treatment restores the balance of the Chi and yin/yang force, which promotes health and healing.

The twelve basic or master meridians and their corresponding organs are also qualified as yin or yang. The yang organs are termed "hollow." The yin organs are said to be "solid." The yang organs transform the body substances and transmit them throughout the body. They also eliminate any unused or unnecessary substances.

9

The yin organs are those which store, produce and regulate the substances of the body. The yin and yang organs are shown below.

Yin (Solid Organs)	Yang (Hollow Organs)
Lung	Large Intestine
Spleen	Stomach
Heart	Small Intestine
Kidney	Bladder
Pericardium	Triple Heater
Liver	Gall Bladder

What You Can Accomplish With Acupressure Massage

You can balance Chi energy in a variety of ways, depending on the body's needs. Stimulating points can release endorphins, the body's pain-reducing substances. Acupressure can also relieve muscle spasms, a primary cause of pain in arthritic conditions. Point stimulation can increase the blood supply to the ailing area, increasing the supply of nutrition and oxygen to the cells. Acupressure can release the body's natural cortisone which reduces swelling. Stimulating certain points will measurably increase antibody production. The increase in immune system activity can reduce infection and relieve low grade fever. Stimulation of certain points has also been shown to influence a variety of immune mediated diseases including canine parvovirus and immune-related skin disorders. Digestion, blood flow, nervous system function, hormone levels and the function of the organs—acupressure can affect all of these.

Chronic as well as acute canine problems respond to acupressure. Generally, a chronic problem will require three to four times as many treatments as an acute problem. The dog experiencing a particular soreness will compensate over time by misusing another part of its body. Both the primary location and the compensating area require treatment. If treatment begins early in the development of the problem, the dog does not have an opportunity to build blockage or injure other parts of its body through compensation.

A Way To Prevent Problems

Traditionally, Oriental doctors were paid only when their patients were healthy. If a patient became ill, the doctor received no payment until full health was restored to the patient. So, you can see the importance of identifying and relieving any Chi energy imbalances in the body before they manifested themselves as disease. You can apply acupressure treatments to prevent health problems. By giving your healthy dog an acupressure treatment two to three times per week, you will help assure that the Chi energy of your dog remains balanced and that your dog can stay in a mode of self-healing.

The ancient Oriental medical practice of acupressure gives you the opportunity to improve your dog's overall well-being and performance. The following chapters detail the acupressure process we have developed for dogs and show you how to perform this treatment on your own dog.

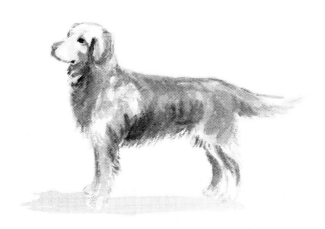

3. THE CANINE MERIDIAN SYSTEM

The pathways that carry Chi throughout the body are the meridians. In Chinese theory these pathways are invisible, but real. The Chi and blood move along the meridians transporting nourishment, strength and healing properties. The meridian system connects and unifies the parts of the body. The Chinese believe it is imperative to maintain the meridians in a balanced state, allowing health and self-healing to occur.

The interior and exterior of the body are connected by the meridian system. As the Chi and blood travel throughout the meridian network their flow and activity can be affected by stimulating "points" along the network. Stimulating acupressure points on the surface of the body affects what goes on inside the body. Because acupressure works to balance the body from outside to inside (via pressure applied at a specific point on the body), it is known as a yang treatment. Herbology, which complements acupressure treatments, is known as a yin activity because it balances the body from the inside out.

Traditional Oriental medicine holds that an imbalance or blockage along a meridian pathway creates disharmony along that meridian. Such an imbalance or blockage can result directly in an imbalance in that meridian's associated organ. For example, an imbalance in the bladder meridian may manifest as a neck ache or an imbalance in the gall bladder meridian may show up as a sciatica problem since these meridians respectively run through these areas of the body.

In dogs as in humans, the meridian system is made up of twelve bilateral major or master meridians. Each of these twelve meridians relates to a specific organ; six yin organs or Zang organs and six yang or Fu organs. In addition to the twelve master meridians, there are eight extraordinary meridians. Two of these, the governing vessel and the conception vessel, are also considered to be master meridians. They are included as master meridians because they have acupressure points on them that are not on any of the other twelve master meridians. The other six extra meridians do not contain any unique acupressure points.

Chi circulates through the meridian system once every 24 hours. The Chi energy is concentrated for approximately two hours in each of the twelve major meridians. During these periods of energy concentration, stimulating association meridian points will generally produce a more powerful result. A flow chart of Chi energy is shown on page 54.

The twelve master meridians are further defined by their association with each other as "sister" or "paired" meridians. Sister meridians have a unique connection with each other. They are the entry and exit points for the flow of Chi energy. Also, one is yin and one is yang. The yang meridian of the pair flows on the top (dorsal) side of the body and the yin meridian of the pair flows along the underside of the body (ventral). Because of these energy and location connections, sister meridians are often both stimulated during an acupressure treatment. If one sister meridian has an excess of energy, the other will show an energy deficiency. Stimulating one or both meridians can alleviate the imbalance. The governing vessel and the conception vessel are the only master meridians that do not have paired counterparts. These two meridians have no direct connection to any of the body's organs and this may be why they are not paired.

This brief introduction to acupressure and the meridian system will help orient you for doing your own acupressure treatment on your canine friends. Important points to keep in mind when working on your dog include:

- An imbalance in Chi energy can cause a state of dis-ease.
- Stimulation of points along meridians can restore balance to Chi energy.
- There are 14 meridians in humans and canines.
- Chi energy is comprised of yin and yang energy.

With these concepts in mind, we can consider the individual meridians, their location, function and important points. Please note that important points are listed for each meridian in the following section. They have been included with each meridian for ease of reference. The next chapter, "Canine Acupressure Points," explains the different types of points and their use.

At the end of this chapter is a diagram of the skeletal system of the dog. When reviewing the location of each meridian, you can use this skeletal system to orient yourself.

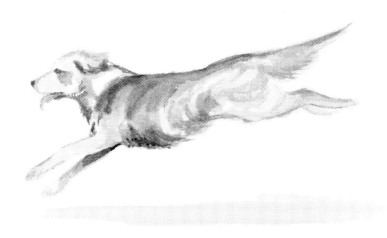

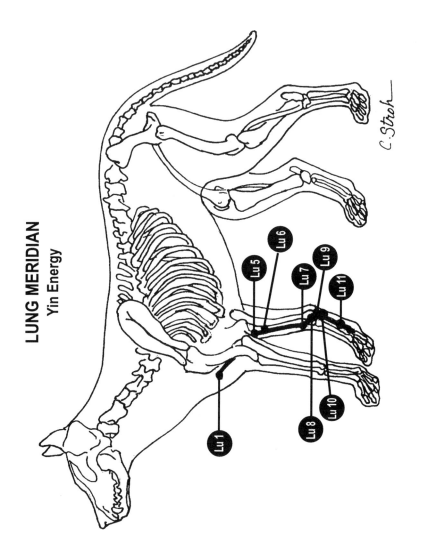

LUNG MERIDIAN
Yin Energy

C. Stroh

Lu 1
Lu 5
Lu 6
Lu 7
Lu 8
Lu 9
Lu 10
Lu 11

Lung Meridian

Sister Meridian:	Large intestine
Maximal Time:	3-5 a.m.
Energy:	Yin

Function: The lung meridian takes in Chi energy from the air and builds resistance to external intrusions. It regulates the secretion of sweat, skin moistening and body hair. This meridian eliminates noxious gases through exhalation. It is also said that the lung meridian rules the Chi, as it regulates the Chi of the entire body governing how much or how little is taken in.

Location: The lung meridian starts at the lung under the shoulder blade. It then travels downward along the inside of the upper arm to the elbow. It continues down the foreleg, passes through the wrist and ends at the dew claw.

Important Points	Type of Point/Use
Lu-1	Relieves fatigue and strengthens the lungs. Use for coughs or asthma.
Lu-5	Main point for all muscular disorders and conditions of excitation. Relieves elbow pain.
Lu-9	Tonification point. Influential point for blood vessels and balances the lungs. Relieves breathing difficulties, clears lungs and relieves wrist pain.
Lu-11	Use for acute emergencies such as respiratory failure, high fever or epilepsy.

Association Point	Alarm Point	Sedation Point
Bl-13	Lu-1	Lu-5
Tonification Point		
Lu-9		

17

LARGE INTESTINE MERIDIAN
Yang Energy

C. Stroh

LI 5
LI 4
LI 3
LI 2
LI 6
LI 1
LI 16
LI 14
LI 13
LI 11
LI 9
LI 15
LI 12
LI 10
LI 8
LI 17
LI 7
LI 18
LI 20

Large Intestine

Sister Meridian:	Lung
Maximal Time:	5 -7 a.m.
Energy:	Yang

Function: The large intestine meridian eliminates stagnation of Chi energy through excretion. It also assists the lung meridian in its functions.

Location: The large intestine meridian starts at the tip of the first toe and travels up the pastern. Here, the meridian crosses to the outside front of the leg where it travels along the foreleg, elbow and upper arm to the shoulder blade. It then travels on the underside of the neck vertebrae under the jaw, curves around the lip and ends at the nose.

Important Points	Type of Point/Use
LI 4	Relieves head, neck, forelimb and shoulder pain. Most important pain reducing point, beneficial for pain in any part of the body. Balances the gastrointestinal system.
LI-10	Use to relieve pain or paralysis of the arm or shoulder. Helps arthritic conditions of the elbow.
LI-11	Tonification point. Relieves constipation and benefits the immune system. Use for arthritic elbow. Often used in the treatment of allergic and infectious disorders.
LI-14	Relieves shoulder tension and relaxes shoulder muscles. Use for relief of stiff neck.
LI-15	Use to relieve arthritis of the elbow and shoulder.

Association Point	Alarm Point	Sedation Point
Bl-25	St-25	LI-2
Tonification Point		
LI-11		

STOMACH MERIDIAN
Yang Energy

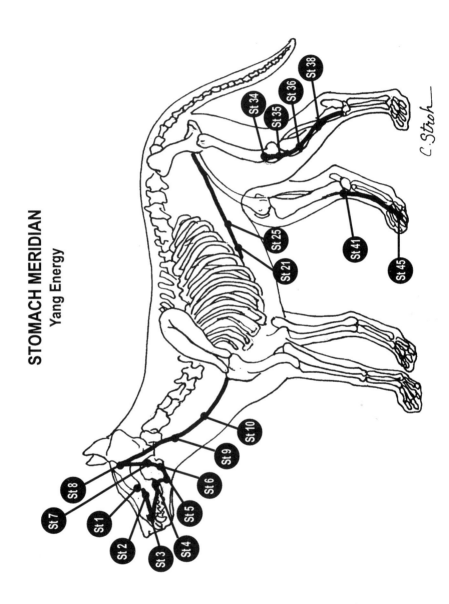

C. Stroh

Stomach Meridian

Sister Meridian :   Spleen

Maximal Time: 7-9 a.m.

Energy: Yang

Function: The stomach meridian relates to the functioning of the stomach and esophagus. It also assists with the reproductive and appetite mechanisms of the body.

Location: The stomach meridian begins under the eye. It descends laterally to the nose and moves along the side of the jawbone. It then turns upward running in front of the ear. From here the stomach meridian runs down below the cervical vertebrae, through the chest, abdomen and loin regions. It runs over the upper thigh muscles to the outer side of the stifle and continues along the center of the front of the hind leg. It travels down the hind leg through the hock and foot and ends at the outside of the second toe.

Important Points	Type of Point/Use
St-1 through 8	Use for disorder of the face, including toothaches and jaw tension.
St-21 & 25	Use for abdominal disorders and to increase circulation in legs. Relieves leg pain and helps all muscles.
St-35	Relieves hind leg joint pain and rheumatism of the feet. Use to relieve pain or arthritis of the stifle.

St-36	General tonification point. Relieves fatigue. Benefits digestion and helps restore the immune system.
St-38 & 41	Use for lameness of the leg, hind limb and joint soreness.
St-45	Relieves nausea, indigestion and abdominal pain.

Association Point
Bl-21
Tonification Point
St -36

Alarm Point
CV-12

Sedation Point
St-45

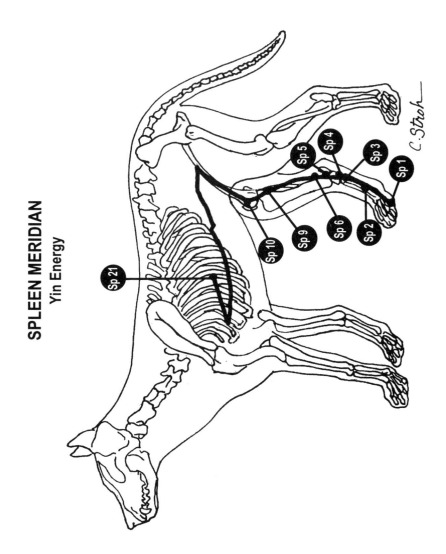

SPLEEN MERIDIAN
Yin Energy

C. Stroh

Sp 21
Sp 5
Sp 4
Sp 3
Sp 1
Sp 10
Sp 9
Sp 6
Sp 2

Spleen Meridian

Sister Meridian :	Stomach
Maximal Time:	9-11 a.m.
Energy:	Yin

Function: The spleen meridian governs the blood. It helps to create blood and assists in maintaining the flow of blood in its proper pathways. The spleen is also said to govern the muscles, connective tissue, flesh and the four limbs, as it originates and carries the Chi to these areas. The movement of the limbs, flesh and muscles is dependent upon a well balanced spleen meridian. This meridian also governs the digestive and fermentation process of the body.

Location: The spleen meridian starts at the outside of the first toe. It travels along the inside of the pastern, over the hock and climbs along the back of the hind leg. It turns forward and crosses the middle of the stifle and upper leg. There it enters the abdominal cavity. It continues along the abdomen, running up to the chest area.

Important Points	Type of Point/Use
Sp-2	Tonification point. Helps relieve constipation.
Sp-4	Regulates and strengthens digestion.
Sp-5	Use for connective tissue weakness and stomach pain.
Sp-6	Junction of the three Yin channels of spleen, kidney and liver. Good point to work to relieve fatigue or weakness. Use for allergic or immune related disorders. Aids in the relief of pelvic limb problems.

Sp-9	Use for hock or pastern problems.
Sp-10	Immune building effects, known as the sea of blood.

Association Point	Alarm Point	Sedation Point
Bl-20	Liv-13	Sp-5
Tonification Point		
Sp-2		

HEART MERIDIAN
Yin Energy

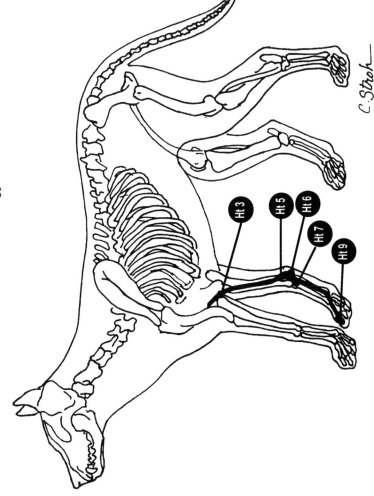

C. Stroh

Ht 3
Ht 5
Ht 6
Ht 7
Ht 9

Heart Meridian

Sister Meridian: Small Intestine
Maximal Time: 11 a.m. - 1 p.m.
Energy: Yin

Function: The heart meridian adapts external stimuli to the internal environment of the body. It is said to govern all other organs. The heart also regulates and circulates blood throughout the body. The heart meridian rules the mental energy or "spirit"of an animal.

Location: The heart meridian runs downward from the chest. It travels along the midline of the upper arm, across the inner elbow and along the midline of the inside of the foreleg. It crosses the wrist and ends at the tip of the inside end of the fourth toe.

Important Points	Type of Point/Use
Ht-3	Use to relieve pain of the elbow.
Ht-5	Use to relieve vision disorders.
Ht-6	Use for behavioral problems. Helps to calm dogs.
Ht-7	Use to calm your dog. Use to help relieve epileptic conditions.
Ht-9	Use to reduce fever. Use for cardio-vascular emergencies. Tonification point.

Association Point	Alarm Point	Sedation Point
Bl-15	CV-14	Ht-7
Tonification Point		
Ht-9		

SMALL INTESTINE MERIDIAN
Yang Energy

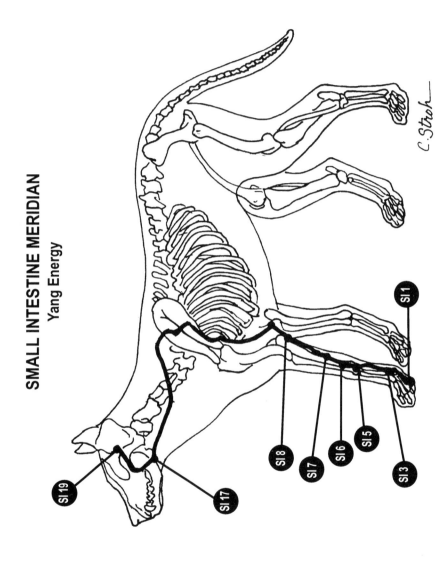

30

Small Intestine Meridian

Sister Meridian:	Heart
Maximal Time:	1-3 p.m.
Energy:	Yang

Function: The small intestine governs the entire body through the digestion and displacement of food.

Location: The small intestine meridian begins on the outside tip of the first toe and runs up along the backside of the pastern and foreleg. It continues up along the back of the upper arm and travels over the shoulder blade. It then travels above the bottom neck vertebrae, turns and travels upward below the remaining neck vertebrae to a point below the jawbone. It then crosses the cheek, runs up to the eye and ends in a point below the ear.

Important Points	Type of Points/Use
SI-3	Use for leg weakness or shoulder pain. Tonification point.
SI-5	Use for colic and muscle spasms of the neck and upper back.
SI-6	Use to relieve stiff neck, forelimb and shoulder pain.
SI-7	Use for shoulder, elbow or foreleg problems.
SI-17	Softens hard muscles and balances the glands.
SI-19	Balances the thyroid gland and relieves excessive ear pressure. Use to relieve facial paralysis.

Association Point	Alarm Point	Sedation Point
Bl-27	CV-4	SI-8
Tonification Point		
SI-3		

BLADDER MERIDIAN
Yang Energy (Dorsal View)

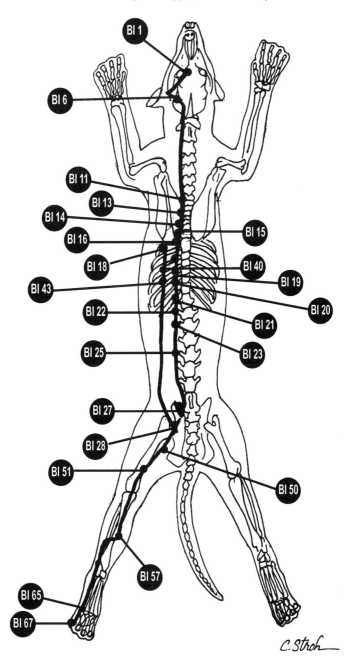

Bl 1
Bl 6
Bl 11
Bl 13
Bl 14
Bl 16
Bl 18
Bl 43
Bl 22
Bl 25
Bl 27
Bl 28
Bl 51
Bl 65
Bl 67
Bl 57
Bl 15
Bl 40
Bl 19
Bl 20
Bl 21
Bl 23
Bl 50

C. Stroh

Bladder Meridian

Sister Meridian:	Kidney
Maximal Time:	3-5 p.m.
Energy:	Yang

Function: The bladder meridian connects to the part of the autonomic nervous system related to reproductive and urinary organs. It purifies the body by means of the elimination of urine. The bladder meridian contains association points for all other meridians.

Location: The bladder meridian begins at a point under the eye and comes over the top of the skull. It then descends along the back of the neck, dividing in two at the base of the shoulder blade. The inner and outer parts of the bladder meridian run parallel to the spine. At the rump, the inner bladder meridian doubles back then returns to its descending flow. The outer portion of the bladder meridian rejoins the inner meridian in the pelvic area. The single meridian now flows down the back of the hind leg and crosses behind the hock. It then turns to the outside at the pastern and continues this flow to the outside of the fourth toe.

Important Points	Type of Point/Use
Bl-6	Activates blood circulation to the head.
Bl-11	Use this point for any type of front leg bone or joint disorder. Helps relieve rheumatoid arthritis and front leg pain. Enhances bone healing.
Bl-13	Lung association point. Use for lung problems including bronchitis or asthma.
Bl-14	Pericardium association point.

Bl-15	Heart association point.
Bl-16	Governing vessel association point.
Bl-18	Liver association point. Use for liver or gall bladder disorders.
Bl-19	Gall bladder association point. Use for liver or gall bladder disorders.
Bl-20	Spleen association point. Useful for calming digestive disorders, vomiting and anemia.
Bl-21	Stomach association point. Use to relieve vomiting.
Bl-22	Triple heater association point. Relieves abdominal pain.
Bl-23	Kidney association point. General arthritis point. Helps relieve back pain. Strengthens immune system.
Bl-25	Large intestine association point. Helps relieve constipation and diarrhea.
Bl-27	Small intestine association point. Relieves indigestion. Use for sciatica pain.
Bl-28	Bladder association point. Helps relieve urinary bladder problems. Use for sciatica pain.
Bl-40	Tonification point. Strengthens the immune system. Use to relieve spasms of the shoulder and upper back.
Bl-43	Use if there is an injury to or pain in the shoulder region.
Bl-50	Use for hip, stifle and hock problems.

Bl-51	Master point of all pain. Use for sacral problems, muscle spasms and cramps of the hind quarters.
Bl-57	Aids in relief of difficult labor.

Association Point	Alarm Point	Sedation Point
Bl-28	CV-3	Bl-65
Tonification Point		
Bl-67		

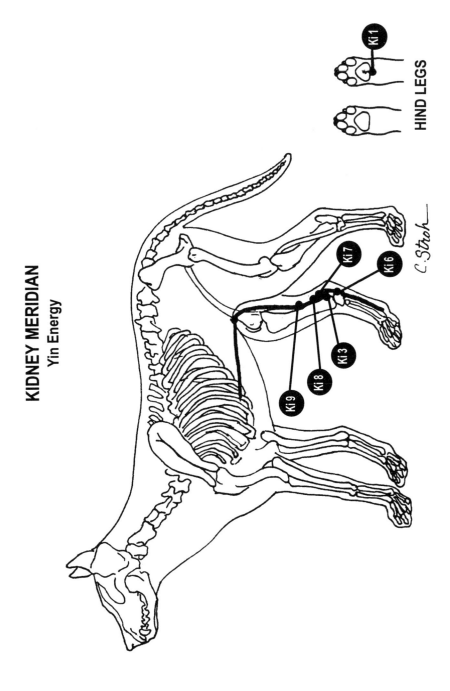

KIDNEY MERIDIAN
Yin Energy

Ki 1
Ki 7
Ki 6
Ki 3
Ki 8
Ki 9

HIND LEGS

C. Stroh

Kidney Meridian

Sister Meridian: Bladder
Maximal Time: 5-7 p.m.
Energy: Yin

Function: The kidney meridian detoxifies the body's blood. It controls the internal secretion of hormones which energize the body. The kidney meridian produces bone marrow, influencing the development and repair of the bones. There is also a close tie between the kidney meridian and the ears.

Location: The kidney meridian begins on the underside of the paw at a point directly behind the center of the communal pad. It emerges on the top side of the toes and runs up the pastern to the hock, where it circles the joint. It then goes up the back side of the hind leg, to the back side of the stifle, climbing upward along the inside of the thigh. The kidney meridian surfaces at the abdomen and runs through the chest to approximately the base of the neck vertebrae.

Important Points	Type of Point/Use
Ki-1	Emergency point for shock, acute seizures and epilepsy. Use only in emergencies since stimulation in non-emergencies can be painful.
Ki-3	Use to help restore the immune system and the reproductive organs.
Ki-6	Regulates hormones. Relieves foot and paw pain.
Ki-7	Stimulate if animal is fatigued. Aids in relief of back pain. Tonification point.

Ki-8

Master point of blood. Regulates the flow of blood to legs. Three Yin channels cross here. Use if there is pain in the legs or hips.

Association Point	Alarm Point	Sedation Point
Bl-23	GB-25	Ki-1
Tonification Point		
Ki-7		

PERICARDIUM MERIDIAN
Yin Energy

C. Stroh

Pe 3
Pe 5
Pe 6
Pe 7

Pe 9
Pe 8

FRONT LEGS

Pericardium Meridian

Sister Meridian:	Triple Heater
Maximal Time:	7-9 p. m.
Energy:	Yin

Function: The pericardium meridian controls nutrition and supplements the heart meridian in blood circulation.

Location: The pericardium meridian begins in the chest cavity near the heart. It surfaces at the elbow, it then runs down the foreleg through the bones of the foot and toes.

Important Points	Type of Point/Use
Pe-3	Use to improve general circulation and depression. Relieves stomach tension.
Pe-5 & 6	Balances the internal organs and relieves wrist pain.
Pe-8	Use to relieve stomach and intestinal spasms.

Association Point	Alarm Point	Sedation Point
Bl-14	CV-17	Pe-7

Tonification Point

Pe-9

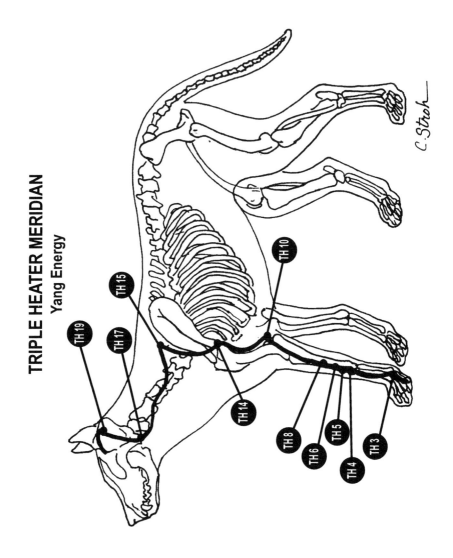

TRIPLE HEATER MERIDIAN
Yang Energy

TH 19
TH 17
TH 15
TH 10
TH 14
TH 8
TH 6
TH 5
TH 4
TH 3

C. Stroh

42

Triple Heater Meridian

Sister Meridian: Pericardium
Maximal Time: 9-11 p.m.
Energy: Yang

Function: The triple heater meridian circulates energy through the entire body. It enhances the function of the lymphatic system and supplements the functions of the small intestine meridian.

Location: Beginning at the outside tip of the 4th toe, the triple heater runs over the top of the toe and foot bones. It runs up the middle of the foreleg to the elbow. It then travels up the backside of the upper arm, crossing at the bottom of the shoulder blade, then runs up the spine of the shoulder blade. The triple heater travels up the neck vertebrae and ends at the back of the ear.

Important Points	**Type of Point/Use**
TH-3	Tonification point.
TH-4	Relieves wrist discomfort such as tendinitis, rheumatism and arthritis.
TH-5	Use for rheumatic conditions. Helps ease tendinitis, regulates and relaxes the body.
TH-6	Use in colic. Affects constipation.
TH-8	Connecting point of three Yang meridians. This is a shoulder, neck and forelimb release point.
TH-10	Sedation point. Use for elbow and forelimb soreness or sprains.
TH-14	Shoulder lameness or soreness.
TH-17	Use for ear problems.

Association Point	Alarm Point	Sedation Point
Bl-22	CV-5	TH-10
Tonification Point		
TH-3		

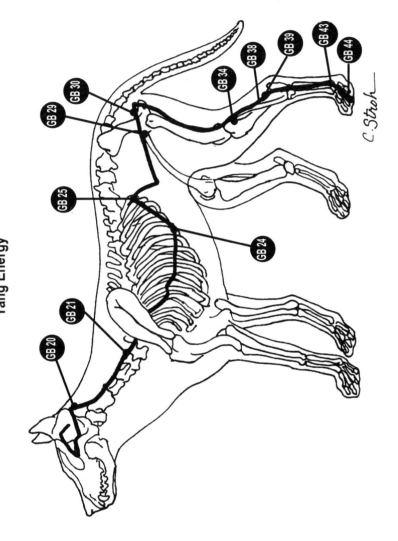

GALL BLADDER MERIDIAN
Yang Energy

GB 20
GB 21
GB 25
GB 29
GB 30
GB 34
GB 38
GB 39
GB 43
GB 44
GB 24

C. Stroh

44

Gall Bladder Meridian

Sister Meridian: Liver
Maximal Time: 11 pm-1 am
Energy: Yang

Function: The gall bladder balances body energy by regulating the internal hormones and secretions and it distributes nutrients throughout the body. The gall bladder rules decisions. Excessive gall bladder Chi may be shown as anger, whereas timidity or shyness are a result of insufficient gall bladder Chi.

Location: The gall bladder meridian starts at the outer corner of the eye. It circles the ear and crosses back and forth on the side of the head then curves behind the ear and flows down the neck vertebrae. It enters the chest cavity and flows through the abdomen. At the pelvic area it follows down the side of the hind leg. It crosses in front of the hock, over the foot and toe bones and ends at the side of the tip of the second toe.

Important Points	Type of Point/Use
GB-20	Alleviates head and neck pain.
GB-21	Relieves shoulder pain. Benefits the shoulder and softens tense muscles. Use for shoulder arthritis.
GB-24	Alarm point for the gall bladder. Use to relieve stomach indigestion and disorders.
GB-25	Use for kidney disorders or problems with water metabolism.
GB-29	Use for all disorders of joints, especially the large joints.

GB-30	Use for sciatica problems and hip dysplasia. Relaxes the tendons and restores joint mobility.
GB-34	Influential point for the muscles and tendons as it relaxes the muscles of the hindquarter. Relieves stifle pain.
GB-39	Influential point for building bone marrow.

Association Point	Alarm Point	Sedation Point
Bl-19	GB-24	GB-38
Tonification Point		
GB-43		

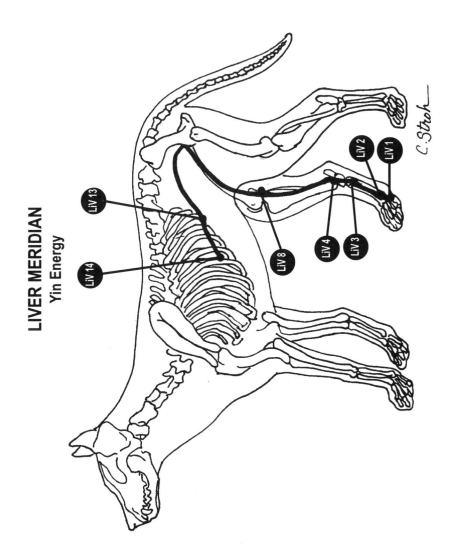

LIVER MERIDIAN
Yin Energy

LIV 13
LIV 14
LIV 8
LIV 4
LIV 3
LIV 2
LIV 1

C. Stroh

Liver Meridian

Sister meridian:	Gall Bladder
Maximal Time:	1-3 a.m.
Energy:	Yin

Function: Has three major functions. First, the liver adjusts and smoothes the movement and flow of Chi energy throughout the body. The liver regulates the secretion of bile, and third, it rules the proper movement of all tendons, ligaments and even some of the body's muscles. Additionally, the liver stores energy and nutrients for physical activities, maintains physical energy through blood detoxification and builds resistance against disease.

Location: The liver meridian begins at the tip of the dew claw and runs up the toes and pastern along the backside of the hind leg and stifle. It continues along the middle of the femur to the pubic region. There it enters the abdomen and passes into the lower chest cavity.

Important Points	Type of Point/Use
Liv-2	Relieves diarrhea and nausea. Calming point. Helps relieve colic.
Liv-3	Invigorates and clears the meridian system.
Liv-4	Relieves pain. Use for colic or stomach upset.
Liv-8	Tonification point. Relieves hock pain.

Association Point	Alarm Point	Sedation Point
Bl-28	Liv-14	Liv-2
Tonification Point		
Liv-8		

49

CONCEPTION VESSEL MERIDIAN
Yin Energy (Ventral View)

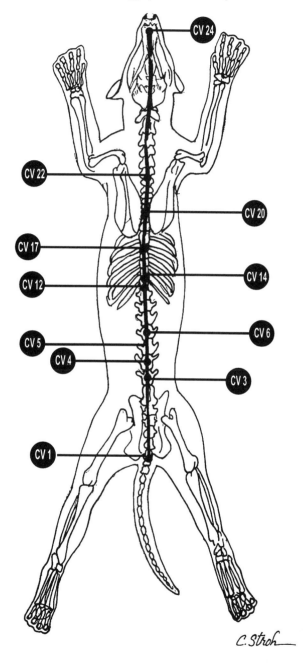

C. Stroh

Conception Vessel Meridian

Sister Meridian: None

Maximal Time: None

Energy: Yin

Function: This meridian controls contractions of the smooth muscles. It is the main source of inherited energy. It is said to control the six Yin meridians and the alarm points. This meridian also influences the genital organs.

Location: The conception vessel begins in the pelvic cavity. It ascends along the midline of the abdomen, chest and throat to the lower jaw. It then penetrates internally to the lips and ends at the mid point of the lower jaw.

Important Points	Type of Points/Use
CV-3	Use to relieve incontinence.
CV-4	Relieves impotence and strengthens the reproductive system.
CV-6	General tonification point. Use for tired or lethargic animal. Helps strengthen the hindquarters.
CV-12	Harmonizes the stomach and relieves stress. Use to relieve vomiting.
CV-14	Reduces heart or stomach stress. Helpful in behavioral problems.
CV-17	Use to activate the flow of Chi energy. Use to help calm the animal.
CV-20	Use to help asthmatic conditions or bronchitis.
CV-22	Strengthens the brain and regulates the lungs and throat.

GOVERNING VESSEL MERIDIAN
Yang Energy (Dorsal View)

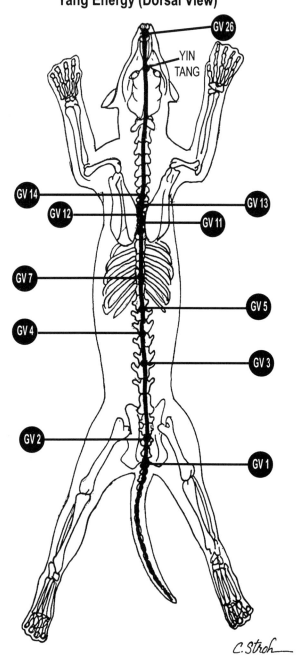

GV 26

YIN
TANG

GV 14

GV 13

GV 12

GV 11

GV 7

GV 5

GV 4

GV 3

GV 2

GV 1

C.Stroh

Governing Vessel Meridian

Sister Meridian: None

Maximal Time: None

Energy: Yang

Function: This meridian is the confluence of all Yang meridians. It has an important governing and controlling role over the other Yang meridians. This meridian helps to coordinate and harmonize all regions of the body and organs. The governing vessel is closely related to the central nervous system.

Location: The governing vessel starts at the tip of the tail. It follows the spinal column along the back to the tip of the nose.

Important Points	Type of Points/Use
GV-1 & 2	Use for constipation or diarrhea.
GV-3, 4 & 5	Use for rheumatism or sprains of the loin area. Use GV-3 to relieve or adjust female reproductive disorders.
GV-7	Use to improve appetite.
GV-11, 12, 13 & 14	Use for shoulder sprains or front leg lameness including arthritic conditions.
GV-26	Use for specific emergencies including shock, collapse, heatstroke or seizures.
GV-Yin-Tang	Use for calming the dog.

Association Point
     Bl-16

DIRECTIONAL AND TIME FLOW
OF CHI ENERGY ALONG THE MERIDIANS

Yin Meridians   **Yang Meridians**

Lung Meridian ━━━━━━ Large Intestine Meridian
3 - 5 AM   5 - 7 AM

Spleen Meridian ━━━━━━ Stomach Meridian
9 - 11 AM   7 - 9 AM

Heart Meridian ━━━━━━ Small Intestine Meridian
11 AM - 1 PM   1 - 3 PM

Kidney Meridian ━━━━━━ Bladder Meridian
5 - 7 PM   3 - 5 PM

Pericardium Meridian ━━━━━━ Triple Heater Meridian
7 - 9 PM   9 - 11 PM

Liver Meridian ━━━━━━ Gall Bladder Meridian
1 - 3 AM   11 PM - 1 AM

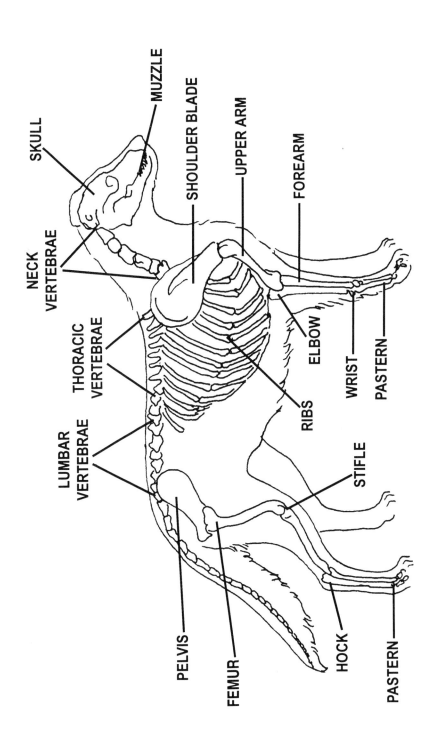

SKULL
MUZZLE
SHOULDER BLADE
UPPER ARM
FOREARM
NECK VERTEBRAE
THORACIC VERTEBRAE
ELBOW
WRIST
PASTERN
LUMBAR VERTEBRAE
RIBS
STIFLE
PELVIS
FEMUR
HOCK
PASTERN

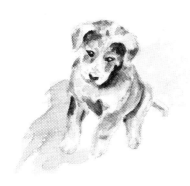

4. CANINE ACUPRESSURE POINTS

Acupressure points are the gateways to the 14 meridians. They are located along each meridian and at other specific points on the body. At the acupressure points, Chi energy flows close to the surface of the body, allowing you to manipulate that energy efficiently by using acupressure techniques. In total, there are over 350 meridian points and over 250 non meridian points.

In dogs, as in humans, the therapeutic value of a point has to do with the meridian on which it is located. Stimulating points on the stomach meridian will benefit the stomach. Points on the same meridian have common values and distinct properties and effects. You can stimulate points located on the head, face and trunk to treat disorders in those areas. You can use points below the elbow, pastern and stifle to treat disorders in other parts of the body. See the meridian charts in the preceding chapter for specific point values and use.

Acupressure points are either permanent—existing at all times— or interim—appearing only during a pathological or disease state. Oriental practitioners have separated the permanent points into various categories based on their use, effect or location. This section describes the points and the categories in which they are grouped.

• **Association Points** Each meridian has an association point which is located on the bladder meridian. These points correspond to individual meridians and may be stimulated to affect that meridian. The meridian and its association point are shown below.

Meridian	Assoc. Point	Meridian	Assoc. Point
Lung	Bl-13	Spleen	Bl-20
Pericardium	Bl-14	Stomach	Bl-21
Heart	Bl-15	Triple Heater	Bl-22
Governing Vs	Bl-16	Kidney	Bl-23
Liver	Bl-18	Large Intestine	Bl-25
Gall Bladder	Bl-19	Small Intestine	Bl-27
		Bladder	Bl-28

The association points are believed to transmit the Chi energy to the associated organ. Because of this property, we recommend their stimulation in most acupressure treatments.

• **Alarm Points** These points are located on the surface of the abdomen with one alarm point connected to each of the internal organs. These points will be tender when their related organ/meridian is distressed. The alarm points and corresponding meridians are shown below.

Meridian	Alarm Point	Meridian	Alarm Point
Lung	Lu-1	Bladder	CV-3
Large Intestine	St-25	Kidney	GB-25
Stomach	CV-12	Pericardium	CV-17
Spleen	Liv-13	Triple Heater	CV-5
Heart	CV-14	Gall Bladder	GB-24
Small Intestine	CV-4	Liver	Liv-14

• **Sedation Points** Located along a meridian line, sedation points are generally warm to the touch and slightly protruding. Stimulating these points disperses blocked energy and begins energy rebalancing. The sedation points of each meridian are shown below.

Meridian	Sedation Pt.	Meridian	Sedation Pt.
Lung	Lu-5	Bladder	Bl-65
Large Intestine	Ll-2 & 3	Kidney	Ki-1 & 2
Stomach	St-45	Pericardium	Pe-7
Spleen	Sp-5	Triple Heater	TH-10
Heart	Ht-7	Gall Bladder	GB-38
Small Intestine	SI-8	Liver	Liv-2

• **Tonification Points** These points are located along a meridian line. Usually these are cool to the touch. If you stimulate one of these points you increase the energy flow to it and begin energy rebalancing. The tonification points are shown below.

Meridian	Tonification Pt.	Meridian	Tonification Pt.
Lung	Lu-9	Bladder	Bl-67
Large Intestine	Ll-11	Kidney	Ki-7
Stomach	St-36	Pericardium	Pe-9
Spleen	Sp-2	Triple Heater	TH-3
Heart	Ht-9	Gall Bladder	GB-43
Small Intestine	SI-3	Liver	Liv-8

Acupressure points do not necessarily have a particular physical shape, rather they are best identified by physical landmarks on the dog's body and by your developing a "feel for the energy." Anyone can develop this "feel." It is a matter of quieting ourselves and becoming receptive to the subtle energies of our companions.

5. CASE STUDIES

This chapter will introduce you to some of the dogs that have come to us for acupressure massage. Nathan, Buck, Retta and the others vary in age, breed and function but they represent physical problems any dog, even your own, may develop. Arthritis, bursitis, shoulder soreness and problems associated with old age are conditions owners can treat successfully with acupressure.

As you read the case studies, here are two important things to keep in mind. First, acupressure massage gives you the opportunity to take an active role in both keeping your dog healthy and healing him if he is ill or injured. Second, acupressure massage does not replace but complements more familiar kinds of veterinary treatment. Veterinarians frequently recommend acupressure massage for dogs after the limits of traditional treatment have been reached.

Owners can think of acupressure massage as an additional means of treatment to try when traditional methods have not been wholly satisfactory. But acupressure treatment should never be regarded as a cure-all. Dog owners should not turn to it expecting miracles. Some dogs cannot return to full functioning even with the best efforts of veterinary medicine and acupressure massage. What acupressure treatment can accomplish is to make each dog more comfortable and more mobile.

Just as acupressure massage can play a role in bringing about the recovery of an ill or injured dog, it can help prevent injury in a well dog. A relaxed and supple dog is a dog well prepared to meet the demands of working, showing or performance sports. Similarly, a relaxed companion dog is more comfortable in his daily routines. For this reason, any dog owner may wish to make acupressure massage a part of his/her dog's regular care routine.

Finally, owners who use acupressure treatment find there is an unexpected benefit. During the treatment, owners themselves enjoy a few quiet and relaxed minutes. They focus their attention completely on the dog. And the owner and dog seem to develop more trust and understanding than they had before. The owner has a chance to exchange the gifts of time and healing attention with the companion whose whole life celebrates those things.

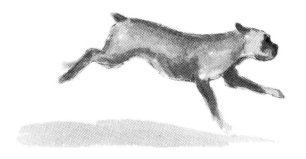

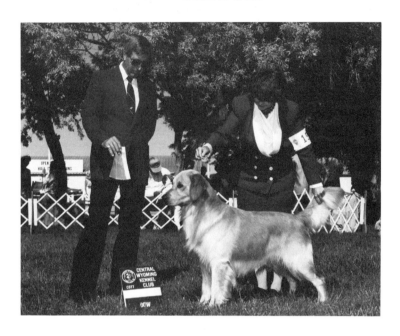

Nathan, an 18 month old Golden Retriever, is a successful show dog and companion of his owner, Sue. His winning record is due in large part to his smooth, bold movement and sweeping stride. Injured while romping with Sue's other dogs, Nathan's continuing pain and his failure to recover led Sue to try acupressure treatment as a possible remedy.

Sue reported that Nathan's injury occurred when he collided with one of her other dogs, about four weeks prior to our seeing Nathan. Following the incident, Nathan was unable to move properly. Both front and rear movement were affected. He could not extend his left front shoulder evenly, nor could he use his hind legs properly.

Sue could demonstrate Nathan's loss of mobility by gently stretching his front legs. The right front leg was clearly more flexible and mobile than the left one.

We found that Nathan's left shoulder was quite tender, as was his back, especially in his right hip and hind leg. Nathan's shoulder injury had strained the other muscles, causing them to become sore. Termed "referred pain", this kind of strain is common with muscular injuries. One set of muscles—the shoulder muscles in Nathan's case—can't do its job so other muscles are forced to compensate.

Our work on Nathan began with the bladder meridian. Once we began to free the flow of energy through his body, we worked on points in his left shoulder and front legs. The points are located on the large and small intestine meridians, and the lung and heart meridians. Nathan adjusted quickly to the massage and relaxed as we worked on him.

As the points on Nathan's shoulder became less sensitive, we moved again to his back and the bladder meridian. After completing this first acupressure massage, we took Nathan outside where we could watch him move. Sue remarked on the improvement she saw. Nathan's fluid stride had returned, he extended his front legs more evenly and his hind legs tracked more correctly.

During a second treatment we worked the bladder meridian points with increased pressure. We then began working the meridians on Nathan's hindquarters, including the liver, gall bladder, kidney and spleen meridians. Here we found several points (jitsu points) that were sensitive and somewhat warm to the touch. Although these points were sensitive, they released easily with gentle pressure.

After completing the work on Nathan's hindquarters and releasing the Chi energy there, we returned to his front legs and shoulder. Here we found the previously highly sensitive shoulder points could now accept increased pressure.

We worked along the bladder meridian once more, then completed the point work by "closing" Nathan. Finally we did a few front leg stretches on Nathan and gently checked his range of motion. We taught Sue to do the treatments. Our suggestions for her included several front leg stretches she could use on alternate days of massaging. Sue maintained this routine for a week and now does the massage on an "as needed" basis.

We saw Nathan three more times, each visit approximately two weeks apart. The acupressure treatments we gave were similar to those described above. At each session we saw fewer sensitive points in both the shoulder and hindquarter areas.

It's been a year since we worked on Nathan. He resumed his career as a show dog, reclaiming the success he had before his injury. Sue comments often on how well he moves and how much he enjoys his acupressure treatments.

BURSITIS
D. J. AND WANDA

D.J. was brought to us by client referral. A friend whose show dog had been helped by acupressure suggested Wanda come to us. D. J. is a 5 year old English Setter. She has excellent breeding and had been performing well in the ring until an unexplained injury put her career on hold.

After the injury Wanda showed D.J. unsuccessfully. She was literally laughed out of the ring. Pessimistic and skeptical, Wanda brought D.J. to us in the late winter.

When D.J. moved, it was obvious that she was "off" in the right front leg. Wanda's veterinarian had taken x-rays but found no identifiable bone problems in D.J.'s legs. He explained her condition as a bursitis of either the shoulder or elbow. With this in mind, we began treatment on D.J., concentrating our work in the area of her neck, right front leg and opposite left hind leg.

We found reactive points on her front legs and shoulders on the gall bladder, heart, small intestine, lung and large intestine meridians. We worked these meridians, balancing the Chi energy flow by releasing blockages and drawing energy to deficient areas. D.J. responded to the treatment by stretching her hind legs, licking and yawning excessively.

We taught Wanda to do the acupressure treatment, showing her the meridians and specific points to work. Wanda continued doing the acupressure work on her own, returning for a session with Marie once a month. Her monthly visits were scheduled as closely as possible to her next show.

Wanda and D.J. went to shows during that spring and summer and D.J. won. By the end of the summer she was awarded her championship. D.J. and Wanda continue to do well. D. J. has started a new career as a brood bitch, whelping several competitive litters.

ARTHRITIC CONDITION
RETTA AND BILL

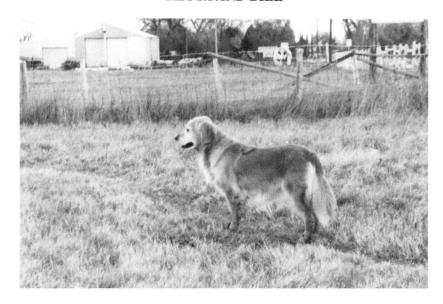

Retta is a 10 year old Golden Retriever. The favorite companion of her owner, Bill, Retta is suffering from arthritis of the hips and shoulders as she ages. She can go up and down steps only with difficulty. Even lying down and moving slowly from place to place is an uncomfortable effort for Retta.

· Bill did not want to believe that Retta's pain had no remedy. He values her companionship and his memories of her as a young, athletic dog, winning her championship and obedience titles. She also produced, in a few, carefully planned litters, puppies who became champions. Bill felt he owed it to Retta to relieve her pain.

For our first session with Retta we worked along the bladder meridian over her body and down the rump on both sides. We found reactive points in the shoulder, hip and stifle areas. In arthritic conditions it is important to work all points around the joints. We did this on Retta's left and right sides. Her condition required that we work points and increase pressure as she allowed, for a period of 10 to 20 seconds.

For the hind quarters we worked the bladder, gall bladder, liver, stomach and kidney meridians. We worked the point designated as "gall bladder 30" several times as it is known to improve joint mobility. We also worked meridian points 36, 38 and 41 on the stomach to stimulate relief for joint soreness.

Retta was somewhat wary of the treatment at first. Slowly she relaxed into the treatment. She reacted to acupressure with excessive yawning, often a sign of low level discomfort, muscle spasms and panting.

We taught Bill a thorough acupressure treatment routine and suggested he massage Retta every other day for 10 days. After that he was to massage her on an "as needed" basis. Bill performs the massage faithfully. He reports that the massages give Retta a significant measure of relief from the pain of her arthritis.

NEUROLOGICAL DYSFUNCTION
BUCK AND BARBARA

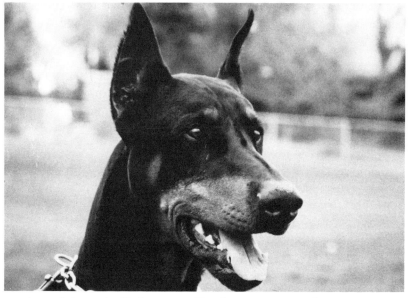

An adult male Doberman, Buck came to us for acupressure treatment while under treatment for a terminal illness. Barbara, Buck's owner, previously sought acupressure treatments for one of her horses. Impressed with the changes in the performance of her jumper, she hoped acupressure massage could make this good dog more comfortable.

Buck was being seen by an area veterinarian and had subsequently been referred to Colorado State University School of Veterinary Medicine (CSU), for further examination. CSU found that Buck had a cancerous brain tumor located behind his left eye. Buck received a series of laser treatments to shrink the tumor and medication aimed at reducing the severity of seizures he was experiencing as a side effect of the laser treatments.

Buck's traditional veterinary medical treatments continued during the time we worked on him.

When Buck came for his first massage, Barbara had to lift him from the car. He stood and walked only with her assistance.

We directed our treatment efforts at releasing Buck's cramped and spastic muscles and at relieving areas of pain. We began Buck's treatment by working the bladder meridian. This begins behind the eye and runs the length of the body, then down the hind legs. We found many reactive points, particularly on the neck, shoulder, barrel and hip areas. The points that were warm to the touch (jitsu points), we worked lightly for three to five seconds. We increased pressure as Buck would allow. We found cool areas (kyo points) on Buck's hips and hind legs and on the bladder, liver and gall bladder meridians. We worked these for as long as two minutes.

Buck's first massage lasted over an hour. His improvement was quite dramatic. After the treatment he got up by himself and walked back to the car without help from Barbara. He was able to water a shrub on the way to the car, something he had not been able to do in proper male fashion for some time.

We taught Barbara to give an acupressure treatment. She continued the work on her own every other day, bringing Buck back to us for a massage every 10 to 14 days. Between treatments, Buck maintained mobility, and comfort levels and reduced severity of seizures. His cancer advanced, however, and Buck was put to rest about four months after treatment began.

Barbara found some comfort in knowing that the massages she gave made Buck's last months less painful. We were proud to be part of that accomplishment.

ZONKER, JEFF AND JANET
CONDITIONS OF OLD AGE

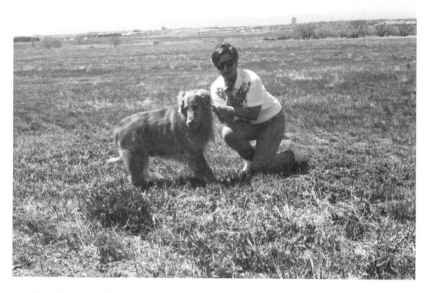

Zonker, an 11 year old male Golden Retriever, came to us after his owners had taken him to their veterinarian. Typical of many older dogs, Zonker was experiencing difficulty in getting up and lying down. His movement in this process was very stiff, he would whine in discomfort and then take shortened steps. Zonker was also a bit overweight and under exercised.

The veterinarian recommended putting Zonker on steroids and anti-inflammatories to lessen his discomfort. Janet and Jeff were aware of the possible side effects of such drugs and, as we had worked on several of Janet's horses with good results, she gave us a call.

In our first session with Zonker we asked him to lie on his side while we worked the bladder, gall bladder, kidney and liver meridians on his back and hindquarters. Zonker was reactive on the bladder meridian on points around the hips. While working these points he displayed reactions of excessive panting and muscle spasms. We then worked the front leg meridians including the lung, large and small intestine, triple heater and heart meridians. There were just a few reactive points along these meridians. We returned our point work to the hindquarters running the same meridians as before. The reactions showed by Zonker had diminished in intensity on the second run. We did the same work on Zonker's other side.

Upon completion of our work Zonker was able to get up and move around in comfort. We showed Janet and Jeff the points to work on Zonker and advised they give him a treatment every other day for one week and then on an "as needed" basis. We also discussed a weight reduction plan for Zonker, as well as an increase of exercise for him.

Janet and Jeff returned for two more sessions with Zonker. At this time his owners continue to give Zonker maintenance treatments one to two times per week. He is given aspirin several times a week and has not been put on any other medications. Zonker's owners have also trimmed his weight and have been diligent about following his exercise program.

6. THE CANINE ACUPRESSURE TREATMENT

As important and beneficial an acupressure treatment can be to your dog, of equal importance is your frame of mind or intent when giving the treatment. Animals are amazingly adept at understanding body language and energy sensations—their survival often depends on this ability. Before beginning an acupressure treatment we suggest owners and practitioners assess their dog's needs and follow the pretreatment exercises detailed below.

PRETREATMENT PRACTICES

You can prepare to give a massage

- by clearing the days activities from your mind,
- by getting in touch with your own Chi energy, and
- by focusing your energy on your dog.

Here are some simple techniques that will help you to accomplish these goals.

GETTING IN TOUCH WITH YOUR CHI ENERGY

Sit quietly for several moments and clear the day's activities from your mind. Allow yourself to release distracting thoughts from your mind like clouds floating out of view. Breathe in the Chi from the air and feel it move through your lungs and down into your abdomen. Hold the Chi in your abdomen for several seconds and feel its balancing and healing properties. Exhale and follow the vibration of your breath as it moves across the room. Repeat this exercise for 10 to 15 breaths. Finally, focus your energy on your dog, feel your love for your dog and remember the fun you have had with him.

INTRODUCING YOURSELF TO THE DOG

If you are working on a dog that does not know you, or even one that does, it is always best if you "introduce" yourself to him before starting the acupressure treatment. The introduction is just normal touching and talking to the dog. Pet the dog lightly, stroking his back, neck and ears. Taking a few moments to let the dog acquaint himself with you and be comfortable with you will minimize stress to the dog and yourself. We don't recommend offering treats as a way of introduction; it often serves only to distract the dog.

USING A HELPER

If you are working on a dog that is not yours, it helps to have the owner present, more to reassure than to restrain. If the dog is in pain, it is always best to have the owner present. The owner's presence gives the dog confidence and allows treatment to progress without incident. The helper can also watch for the dog's responses to the treatment.

WHERE TO DO A TREATMENT

When you start an acupressure treatment, choose a location familiar to the dog. Be sure he is comfortable in these surroundings. You may work either outside or indoors. We find that working indoors, especially for the first few treatments, is less distracting for your dog and ultimately for you. It can be difficult to give an acupressure treatment to a tense or squirmy dog, so if your dog has a special place, like the rug beside your bed or a sunny spot in the living room, work there.

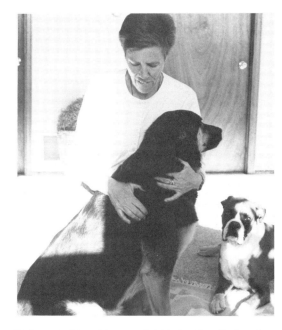

Here Marie works "Bruno" in a comfortable location. Having other dogs around may also be comfortable for the dog you're working on.

Allow your dog either to stand while being given a treatment or to lie down, whichever is most comfortable for him. Often a dog will start the treatment standing, sit down and then lie down as he relaxes and begins to receive the benefit of the acupressure treatment.

WORKING ON A LARGE OR SMALL DOG

The treatment principles of acupressure are the same whether you are working on a ninety pound Rottweiler or a five pound Miniature Poodle. You will, however, need to be sensitive to the size and condition of your dog and make adjustments to meet your dog's specific needs. For example, it may be easier and more comfortable for your Dachshund if you hold him in your lap while treating a lower back soreness. For the large dog it is often easier to work the majority of meridians while the dog is standing. For the small dog you will want to be sensitive to the amount of pressure you use while doing point work. One to two pounds of pressure may be the maximum required for your Pekingese as compared to three to five pounds of pressure for your Irish Setter. Just remember to use common sense while doing an acupressure treatment and consider your dog's comfort needs .

LONG HAIRED DOGS

The acupressure treatment can be performed on any breed of dog. Some adjustments in technique and grooming will be helpful, though. First, brush a long haired dog thoroughly before beginning a treatment. This will allow you to feel the energy meridians more easily and give your thumbs more direct access to the skin.

After the dog is brushed, press your fingers through the coat until you feel contact with the skin and locate the meridian. Then, keep your thumbs in contact with the skin when applying pressure to a point. Typically you can glide your fingers along the meridian line without losing contact with the skin. With a long haired dog it is sometimes necessary to take your thumb completely off the dog and then move to the next point, redevelop skin contact and then apply pressure. With a little practice, you will develop a pattern that works for you and your long haired dog.

ACUPRESSURE FOR THE OLDER DOG

Acupressure can particularly benefit the older dog. Arthritis, muscle strains, digestive disorders, old age and other conditions respond well to acupressure. The treatment patterns described in this section readily apply to older dogs. Simply adjust the pressure you use and allow your dog to be comfortable when giving a treatment.

THE FOUR PHASES OF THE ACUPRESSURE TREATMENT

Acupressure treatment has four phases. These phases are opening, point work, closing and meridian stretches. As you do the work of each phase, it is important for you to be relaxed and receptive to your dog. Remember to clear and center yourself. Allow your breathing to become deep and relaxed. This will assist in balancing your dog's Chi and promote its healing benefits.

When you begin the acupressure work, be sure to set aside enough time so that you and your dog are not rushed. As you gain competence you will be able to complete the treatment in less time. Generally it will take twenty minutes to one hour to complete a treatment. The opening will take five to ten minutes, point work ten to thirty minutes, closing five to ten minutes and stretches five to ten minutes.

REACTIONS TO TREATMENT

Your dog may respond to the acupressure massage in various ways. Some reactions such as back hollowing, muscle spasms, excessive licking or yawning, are obvious. As reactions occur, jot them down in a notebook, specifying the phase of treatment in which they occur. For example, "First acupressure treatment produced muscle spasms of the lower back, lasting for 5—10 seconds. Spasms occurred during point work. In the closing phase the muscle spasms recurred, lasting approximately two to four seconds." By doing this you will have an ongoing record of your dog's reactions, changes and progress.

Equally important are the less obvious signs your dog will exhibit. Subtle reactions include changes of facial expression, relaxation of the eye, neck twisting, stretching, chewing, intestinal sounds, changes in breathing rhythm, moving into or away from the point pressure or leg stretching. This is not an exhaustive list of reactions. You should view any behavior unusual for your dog as a reaction. Your list will increase your awareness of your dog's body and its healing process.

You may find that your dog will be tender following an acupressure treatment. Do not be alarmed. It takes 24 hours for Chi energy to cycle throughout the body; therefore, it generally takes 24 to 36 hours for your dog to show improvement.

You can safely give an acupressure treatment to your dog under most circumstances. However, there are certain conditions when you should not give your dog an acupressure treatment.

DO NOT GIVE AN ACUPRESSURE TREATMENT IF:

1. Your dog is pregnant.

2. Your dog has just been fed. Wait three to four hours after he eats before beginning a treatment.

3. Your dog is fatigued from a strenuous walk, run or other exertion. Wait until his breathing returns to normal and he is cooled down.

4. Your dog has just bred or been bred. Wait 12 hours before treating a stud. Before doing a full acupressure treatment on your bitch, determine if she is pregnant. If she is, wait until she delivers before doing a full acupressure treatment.

5. Your dog has a high fever. Call your veterinarian for help.

6. Your dog has an infectious disease. Call your veterinarian for help.

OPENING

"Opening" is the first phase of an acupressure treatment. It introduces the treatment to your dog in a non-threatening and relaxing manner. The opening causes your dog to become aware of its body in preparation for point work. The structured touch of an acupressure treatment is not the same as the petting touch to which it is accustomed. Again, the opening is important as it begins to orient your dog to structured touch.

With your dog in a relaxed position, you are ready to begin the opening. On a dog, an acupressure opening is performed from front to rear and from top to bottom, following the direction of energy flow along the meridian lines. When doing an opening, position the palm in full contact with the dog, using approximately three pounds of pressure. Glide your palm over your dog's body, shaping your hands to the contours of its body. Do not use your fingers. Position the pressure in the heel of your palm and stroke down along the bladder meridian. This technique relaxes the dog and allows you to distinguish differences in your dog's body temperature and muscle tone. It also allows you to feel for surface protrusions or depressions. The ability to feel these differences in temperature and body contour may take some time to develop. That's normal. Just relax and allow your hands to explore your animal's body and its subtle differences.

Do opening from front to rear and top to bottom. Glide your palm over your dog's body. Here Marie opens the bladder meridian.

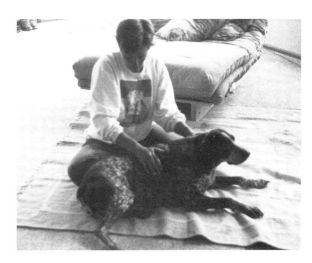

Next, stroke downward from the neck to the top of the shoulders, again from the shoulders to the rump following the bladder meridian.

Then, using firm pressure, stroke from the sacral area, over the rump and down the rear leg to the hock. Repeat the opening procedure two to three times.

When doing an opening watch for signs of sensitivity, areas of heat or coolness, and any reactions from your dog. Also note the different characteristics of the various muscles; for example, rigidity or mushiness, protrusions or depressions. These characteristics may indicate a deficiency or excess of Chi in a meridian and signal that point work is necessary in that area.

REVIEW OF OPENING PROCEDURE

1. Position your dog in a comfortable and familiar location.

2. Place your palm in full contact with the dog.

3. Exert approximately three to five pounds of pressure. Focus the pressure into the heel of your hand, not your fingers.

4. Glide the heel of your hand from front to rear, top to bottom of your dog.

5. Watch for and note reactions or areas of sensitivity.

6. Repeat opening two to three times on both sides.

POINT WORK

Point work stimulates specific points along a meridian line. It is the foundation of acupressure treatment and its second phase. When you stimulate individual points along the meridian lines, you release energy blockages or draw energy to deficient areas. This allows the dog to assist in its own healing process. Canine musculoskeletal ailments respond dramatically to this work.

You may choose any of three methods to do point work.Use the one most comfortable or effective for you and your dog. These methods are the direct pressure thumb technique, the pulsing thumb technique and the circular thumb technique. You may also use a combination of these techniques on your dog during an acupressure treatment.

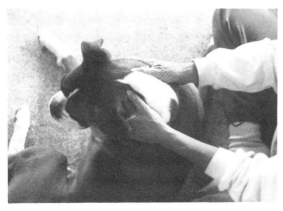

Position ball of thumb at the acupressure point perpendicular to the meridian line. Here Marie begins work on the bladder meridian.

When you do point work, place the ball of your thumb on the acupressure point. Your thumb should be perpendicular to the meridian line on which you are working. As in the opening phase, point work is done from front to rear and top to bottom. Stimulate each point for three to five seconds. It is difficult to state specifically how much pressure should be used. The best procedure is to use gentle pressure at first, approximately two to four pounds, then increase pressure as your dog allows. As shown in the above picture it is best to keep both hands on your dog while giving a treatment. One hand does the point work. The other hand can feel reactions such as muscle spasms and also serves to soothe your dog.

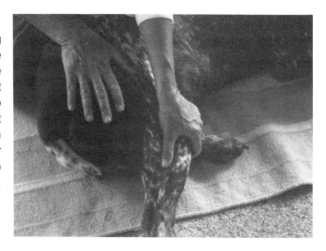

Marie demonstrating the acupressure technique. Here she is using the direct pressure thumb technique. Notice that both hands are on the dog to feel for reactions and to reassure the dog.

Gently put pressure into a point and slowly release out of a point. When stimulating a point, straighten your arm at the elbow and lean into the point with partial body weight. This technique is necessary mostly for large dogs, with smaller dogs you should not need to use body weight. Do not just use your thumbs. Performing the treatment in this manner saves your fingers and wrists from unnecessary fatigue and minimizes any tendency to "jab" at the point. Avoid abrupt movements or changes in pressure. Synchronize your breathing pattern with point stimulation. Breathe out while easing into the point and breathe in while releasing it. Your dog may synchronize its breathing with you after several treatments.

Another method you can use in doing point work is the pulsing thumb technique. This technique is useful to help sedate or tonify points. A light pulsing motion is used to sedate a point while a heavier pulsing motion is used to tonify a point.

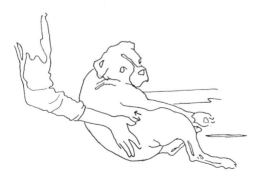

Here Marie demonstrates the "pulsing thumb" technique. Pulsing to the dog's heart rate can enhance point work.

Another acupressure method you can use on your dog is the circular thumb technique. In this method you apply direct pressure to the point with one thumb. Gently ease into the point, applying two to four pounds of pressure. Next, while continuing to apply pressure, rotate your thumb in a circular motion. To tonify or strengthen energy at a point, rotate your thumb in a clockwise motion. To sedate or release energy from a point, rotate your thumb in a counter clockwise motion. Complete three to nine full revolutions. Release gently from the point and move on to the new point and repeat the technique.While using the circular thumb technique keep your free hand on your dog. This constant contact with your dog is comforting to him and helps you feel any muscle spasms, twitching or other reactions to the point work such as heat, cold or sweating.

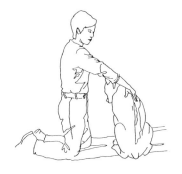

Here Marie demonstrates direct point work. Notice that her thumb is held at a 90° angle to the bladder meridian.

Based on your dog's reaction to the opening, proceed with point work along the meridian lines. Focus on specific areas of energy blockage. A spontaneous pain reaction at any point may indicate a disorder in that particular meridian. Tenderness, revealed by light pressure, indicates that the meridian has an excess of Chi energy. Tenderness, revealed by heavy pressure, identifies an area deficient in Chi energy.

In the opening phase of the treatment, you were asked to feel for depressions or protrusions on your dog. The points which protrude, called "jitsu," indicate areas of excessive energy. The depressed points, called "kyo," show a deficiency of energy.

Jitsu points are warm to the touch. Your dog will react immediately if you stimulate these points. He may move away, retract the limb you are working on or tense and hollow his back. Because jitsu points have an excess of energy they are usually very sensitive to the point work and should be stimulated with light pressure.

When you find a jitsu point stimulate it gently, holding each point for three to five seconds in order to begin releasing the blockage. Points located away from the jitsu area also need to be stimulated to open them and draw the energy excess away from the jitsu point. Work points on the same meridian both above and below the identified jitsu points. This maximizes the release of the blockage at the jitsu points. This procedure begins to balance your dog's energy and is known as a sedation process. The circular thumb technique is particularly beneficial when used to sedate the jitsu or hot points you locate along a meridian. When you stimulate the hot points you will disperse Chi energy away from those points and begin to restore balance to your dog.

Kyo points, or energy deficient areas, are cooler in temperature than the surrounding area. Kyo points require longer stimulation. The best indicator of sufficient point stimulation is a warming of the kyo point. This can take anywhere from 15 seconds to one minute, or longer. When you stimulate the kyo's surrounding meridian points you draw energy and strength into the deficient area and normalize the entire body's energy flow.

With regular acupressure work, you can keep acute or jitsu problems from becoming chronic or more serious ailments. Generally speaking, a chronic ailment in your dog will show up as a kyo condition while an acute ailment will show up as a jitsu condition. A kyo condition might take longer to correct because the dog's healing power is depleted. Patience and strengthening treatments are required for this condition.

CLOSING

The third phase of the acupressure treatment is the closing. It has two purposes. First, closing connects the energy flow between the points stimulated during point work. This reestablishes a more balanced energy flow along the meridian lines. Secondly, the closing work begins repatterning cellular memory. Cellular memory has been described by kinesiologists as the cell's learned response to a chronic stimulus such as pain. The acupressure closing phase replaces the cell's previously learned negative response with a positive one.

You may choose from the three types of closings. Whichever one you choose for your dog, do it twice on each side of your dog to complete the closing.

The first closing technique is the same as the opening phase discussed earlier in this chapter. It is known as the "smooth hand" technique. Position the heel of your hand in full contact with the dog, using approximately five pounds of pressure. Glide the heel of your hand over the dog's body from front to rear, and top to bottom. Remember to focus the weight into the heel of your palm.

The second technique is known as "cupped hand" percussion. Position your hand in a relaxed "pyramid" shape. A side view looks like an "A". When you execute this technique your palm should not make contact with the dog. Remember to keep your wrists relaxed. Use your two hands to alternately strike the body of your dog in a continuously rhythmic motion. If your hands make a bass sound as you strike, you have positioned your hands properly and are keeping your wrists loose. As in the opening, begin the closing at the neck of your dog, moving from front to rear and top to bottom. This closing results in a stimulating yet relaxing finish.

The picture illustrates the "cupped hand" percussion closing technique.

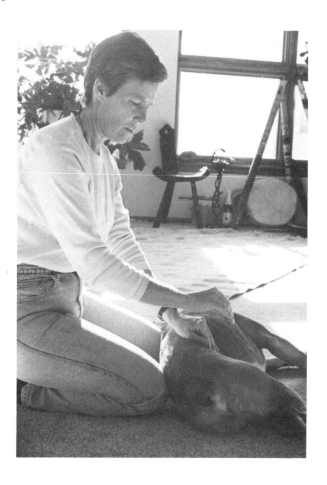

The illustration below shows the third or "rocking hand" type of closing. Use both hands in a light rocking motion. Apply pressure through the palms. Move two to three inches down the dog's body with each rocking movement. Again, the direction of work is from front to rear, and top to bottom. Repeat the closing of your choice two times.

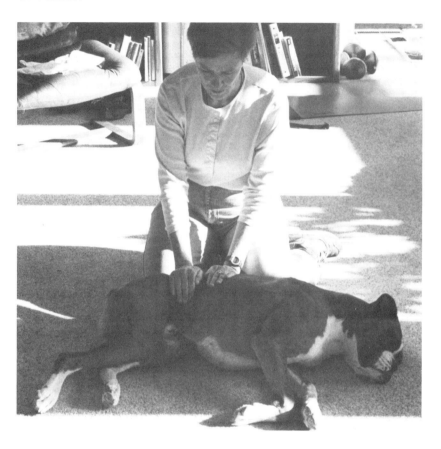

REVIEW OF CLOSING PROCEDURE

1. Choose any one of the three optional closing techniques.

2. Close your dog from front to rear, top to bottom.

3. Repeat closing two times on both sides of your dog.

REVIEW OF OPENING PROCEDURE

1. Position your dog in a comfortable and familiar location.
2. Place your palm in full contact with the dog.
3. Exert approximately two to four pounds of pressure. Focus the pressure into the heel of your hand, not your fingers.
4. Glide the heel of your hand from front to rear, top to bottom of your dog.
5. Watch for and note reactions or areas of sensitivity.
6. Repeat opening two to three times on both sides.

REVIEW OF POINT WORK PROCEDURE

1. Place thumb perpendicular to meridian line.
2. Stimulate point by gently easing into and out of the point.
3. Work points from front to rear, top to bottom.
4. Identify cool and warm areas, stimulate warm areas for three to five seconds, stimulate cool areas for 15 seconds or longer.
5. Watch for and note reactions or areas of sensitivity.
6. Repeat point work on each side of your dog.

REVIEW OF CLOSING PROCEDURE

1. Choose any one of the three optional closing techniques.
2. Close your dog from front to rear, top to bottom.
3. Repeat closing two times on both sides of your dog.

DO NOT GIVE AN ACUPRESSURE TREATMENT IF:

1. Your dog is pregnant.
2. Your dog has just been fed. Wait three to four hours after the dog eats, before beginning a treatment.
3. Your dog is fatigued from a strenuous walk, run or other exertion. Wait until his breathing returns to normal and he is cooled down.
4. Your dog has just bred or been bred. Wait 12 hours before treating a stud. Before doing a full acupressure treatment on your bitch, determine if she is pregnant. If she is, wait until she delivers before doing a full acupressure treatment.
5. Your dog has a high fever. Call for veterinarian help.
6. Your dog has an infectious disease. Call your vet.

7. ACUPRESSURE STRETCHES

The stretches make up the fourth phase of acupressure treatment. These exercises are designed to improve your dog's overall flexibility as well as to improve his well-being and performance. Companion dogs will benefit from these stretches as much as dogs used for show, agility, coursing, herding or sledding. The stretches complement the use of acupressure treatments. These stretches help open certain meridian lines on which the individual acupressure points are located.

The stretches shown in this section can be done singly or in their entirety based on your dog's individual needs. Stretches for specific problems are discussed in Chapter 9. The frequency of stretching is like that for human athletes, with consistency being a major factor in well-being. If you have a show or other competition, do the stretches consistently beforehand. Hurrying through the stretches an hour before show time will do little good.

To ensure maximum benefit and to avoid problems, make all stretching movements slow and fluid, just as you would do in your own stretching routine. As you do the exercises, hold the dog's leg in full extension or flexion with consistent traction—no bouncing. Always return your dog's leg to its original position. Do not allow your dog to pull its leg away. You may need to do the stretches several times until he gets the idea. When first showing him the stretches, he may pull his leg away. If so, go with him and gently show him where you want the leg placed.

The stretches complement the acupressure treatment and they serve four purposes. First, they open the meridians, enhancing the energy flow. Second, they relax and tone muscles, improving suppleness. Third, they increase flexibility, which improves performance and prevents injury. Fourth, they aid in rehabilitative therapy.

As with the acupressure treatment, spend a few minutes grounding and clearing yourself before beginning the stretches. Start slowly with your dog as these movements may be new to him. Also be careful of your own body when doing stretches. Use your entire body, not just your back muscles. For your safety and that of your dog, advance slowly and with caution. When doing the stretches on your own dog, adapt your position to the size of your dog.

FRONT LEG STRETCHES

1. Deltoid and Biceps Stretch

With your dog lying down, grasp the front leg as shown in the photograph. Stretch the leg parallel to your dog's body toward the hind legs. Maintain constant traction. Your dog's shoulder should be extended backwards. Ask your dog to hold the position for a count of ten. Again, if your dog refuses to hold the position, the stretch is beyond its capabilities. Repeat the exercise twice.

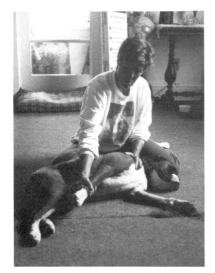

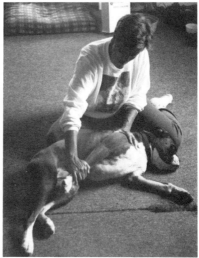

2. Shoulder Extension Stretch

Kneel in front of your dog. Grasp the foreleg below the elbow and at the wrist and lift until the toe is about four inches off the ground. Slowly pull the dog's foreleg toward your chest, asking your dog for a full shoulder extension. Gently place your dog's toe as far in front as it will permit. If your dog holds its leg where you place it, you will know that the stretch was within its capability. If your dog moves its leg backward, it is shifting to a position of comfort, telling you that the stretch was outside its capability. Ask the dog to hold the extension for a count of ten. Repeat exercise two times.

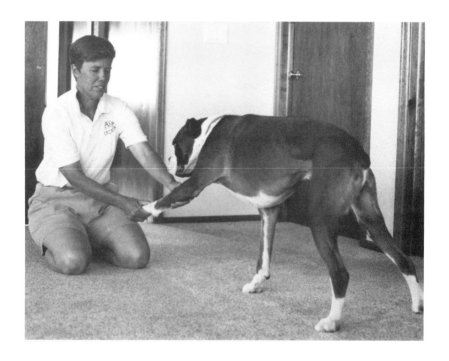

3. Shoulder Rotation Stretch

Kneel in front of your dog, facing its forelegs. Grasp the front leg below the elbow with both hands. Raise the leg to the point of resistance and then lower the leg approximately one inch. Slowly rotate the foreleg in complete circles. Start with small circles and gradually increase the diameter. Reverse the direction of rotation. Rotate the foreleg five times in each direction.

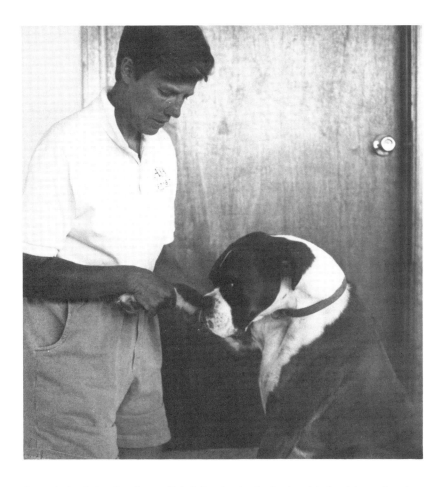

Grasp the leg below the elbow, with both hands raise foreleg to point of resistance, then lower one inch. Rotate slowly and carefully in both directions.

REAR LEG STRETCHES

1. Buttocks Stretch

With your dog lying in front of you, sit at the middle of his back. With your back hand, stabilize your dog's flank. With your front hand grasp your dog's leg below the hock and slowly extend it forward, parallel to his body. Using gentle traction pull the hind leg directly forward, as though your dog were taking a step. Stop when you feel resistance. Hold for a count of ten. Replace the leg to its original position. Repeat exercise twice.

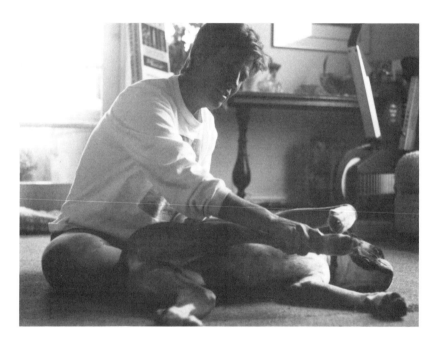

Grasp inside of leg above the hock, support lower leg with outside hand. Direct forward, stop when resistance is felt.

2. Stifle/Pelvis Stretch

With your dog lying in front of you, sit at his hindquarters. With your back hand, gently pick up and stretch his leg in line with his hip in a backward motion. Continue the stretch until the leg is fully extended to the point of resistance. Bring the leg back to a resting position. Repeat the exercise twice.

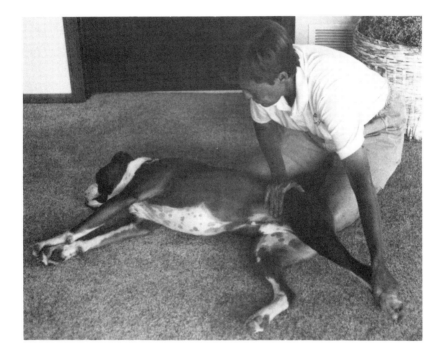

Grasp hind leg and lift one toe about four inches off the ground. Stretch leg in line with body.

3. HIP FLEXION STRETCH

Sitting at the middle of your dog, grasp his leg below the hock with your front hand. Direct the leg towards your body until resistance is felt. Move the leg towards the dog's front feet, then to the rear in a circular motion. Repeat the exercise twice.

Move leg into dog's body.

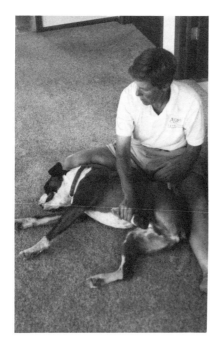

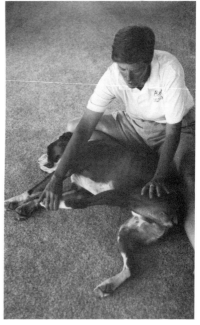

Bring leg forward in gentle movement.

NECK STRETCHES

This exercise improves your dog's neck flexibility and will release areas of tension in his neck.

With your dog sitting if front of you place your hands under his jaw. Gently stretch his head up and back. Repeat exercise 3 times.

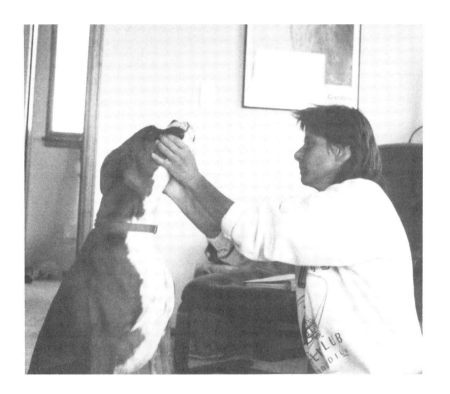

Raise your dog's head gently, stretching the muscles of the neck and chest.

8. ACUPRESSURE MAINTENANCE TREATMENT

Just as acupressure treatments are invaluable for ailing dogs, they also help dogs that are not sick or injured maintain their well-being. Two to four acupressure treatments per week will keep your dog's energy meridians open and balanced. This balanced state of energy flow will improve your dog's overall attitude and will keep minor aches from turning into major ailments. By doing the acupressure stretches two to four times per week, you will increase your dog's suppleness and decrease the possibility of muscle strains.

Many dog owners simply make the acupressure treatment part of their exercise routine. You may either work your dog prior to his daily exercise or after his walk and playtime are complete. Try each with your dog and choose which works best for you.

Before you begin the maintenance treatment, remember to work on your dog in a place familiar to him and where he feels comfortable. Remember also to clear your mind of the day's activities and focus on yourself and your dog. Formulate and communicate your intent to yourself and your dog.

To do the maintenance treatment, open your dog as described in Chapter 6, picking one of the several opening procedures illustrated. Do the opening work from front to back, and top to bottom. Remember to feel for areas of heat or coolness or protrusions or depressions. The opening phase should take between three and eight minutes.

Chapters 8 and 9 present charts, with points to be worked, and a description of the procedure to be completed. After doing several of these treatments it is very likely that you will not need to use the book for guidance. Feel free to explore your dog's energy meridians and work areas you feel need extra attention.

The treatments will be fun for both you and your dog. Enjoy them.

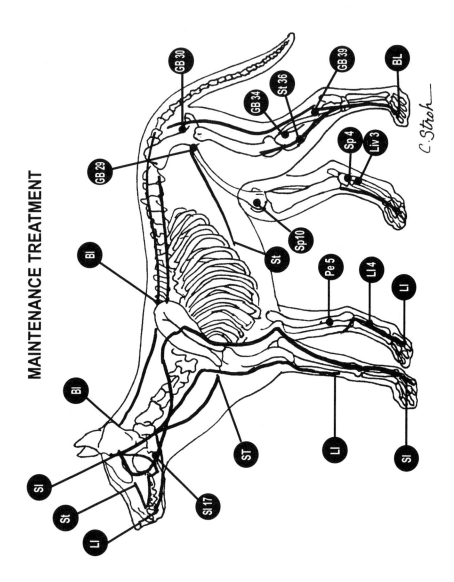

MAINTENANCE TREATMENT

C. Stroh

98

Point Work

1. Stimulate the bladder meridian from the head over the croup and down the hind legs.
2. Stimulate the small intestine meridian from the neck to the bottom of the front legs.
3. Work the gall bladder points as shown.
4. Work the large intestine meridian from below the jaw down both front legs.
5. Work the stomach meridian from below the jaw to the base of the shoulder. Move your hands to your dog's hind legs and begin work on the stomach meridian from the stifle to the pastern.
6. Watch for and note reactions and areas of sensitivity.
7. Close your dog, working from front to rear, top to bottom.

<u>**Important Points**</u>

Bl	Work entire meridian
LI	Work entire meridian, point 4
Liv	3
Pe	5
GB	29, 30, 34 & 39
SI	Work entire meridian, point 17
St	Work entire meridian, point 36

Stretches

1. Do the deltoid and biceps muscle stretch.
2. Do the shoulder rotation stretch.
3. Do the stifle/buttocks stretch.
4. Do the hip flexion stretch.
5. Do the neck stretch.

Frequency

Do the maintenance acupressure treatment two to four times per week.

9. ACUPRESSURE TREATMENT FOR SPECIFIC PROBLEMS

The following pages describe treatments we have developed and used to heal such frequently seen problems as lower back soreness, neck stiffness and hip problems. These treatments are based on our work with show and pet dogs over a period of several years.

Where the owner has been consistent in giving the dog treatments, each dog presented to us has shown significant improvement. The acupressure treatments are not difficult, but they do require regular application. With many canine musculoskeletal ailments, the problems did not appear overnight. By doing the acupressure treatment you may often see dramatic improvement. To maintain the improvement, be consistent with the treatments.

When you do the treatments, do the acupressure work as a unit. Begin with clearing and focusing yourself for work on your dog. Then start with the opening, complete the point work, close your dog and then do the suggested stretches. The first few times you do the treatments, make sure you have enough time and you are not rushed. As you gain competency and efficiency, you will find that the time required to give an acupressure treatment will be cut, perhaps in half. This won't be due to your hurrying through the treatment, but to the increased skill you will have developed in finding the meridians and acupressure points.

Again, we recommend you consult your veterinarian for all canine ailments. Acupressure work is not a substitute for traditional veterinary medicine, but a complement to it.

ARTHRITIC CONDITIONS

Shows Up As
- Specific joint soreness or inflammation
- Difficult or impeded movement of joints
- General discomfort of animal

Refer to drawings on the next two pages for the meridians and points to be worked.

Procedure/Use

To reduce your dog's discomfort from an arthritic condition, work the points on the next two pages. Two drawings are shown, one for front leg and shoulder arthritis and one for back and hindquarter arthritic conditions. If these points are stimulated every other day, they will increase circulation, reduce inflammation and increase joint mobility.

Forequarter Arthritic Condition

Begin by opening your dog as described in Chapter 6. Work the bladder meridian next, giving special attention to bladder points 11 and 23. Next work the gall bladder, large intestine and triple heater meridians. Complete point work by stimulating the stomach meridian, particularly stomach 36, and the the governing vessel meridian. Complete point work on both sides of your dog and then close your dog as described in Chapter 6.

Important Points to be Worked

Meridian	Points	Meridian	Points
LI	4, 10, 11 & 15	Bl	11 & 23
TH	4, 10, & 14	GB	21 & 29
GV	11, 12, 13 & 14	St	36

Frequency

Administer the acupressure treatment every other day until condition improves and then as needed.

ARTHRITIC CONDITION
Forequarter

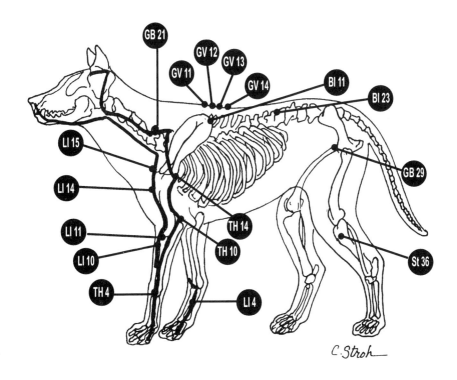

NOTE: See Chapter 3 For Location of Full Meridians

Hind Quarter Arthritic Condition

Begin the treatment by opening your dog as previously described. Begin point work on the bladder meridian, working points 21, 23, 50 and 51 specifically. Next work the stomach meridian, concentrating point work at points 21, 35, 36, 38 and 41. Complete the treatment by working the spleen, kidney, gall bladder and large intestine meridians. Work points on these meridians as noted below. Close your dog, using one of the three methods shown in Chapter 6.

Important Points to be Worked

Meridian	Points	Meridian	Points
St	21, 35, 36, 38 & 41	GB	29, 30 & 34
Bl	21, 23, 50 & 51	Sp	6 & 9
Ki	7 & 8	LI	4 & 11

Frequency

Administer the acupressure treatment every other day until condition improves and then as needed.

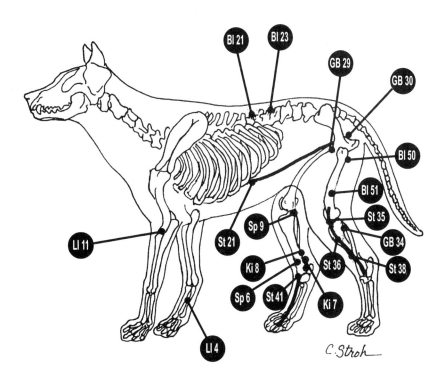

C. Stroh

SHOULDER SORENESS

Shows Up As
- Restricted front leg mobility, shortness of front leg extension
- Off beat cadence at the trot
- Shuffling gait
- Front leg lameness with an offness shown on the opposite hind leg

Refer to drawing on opposite page for meridians and points to be worked.

Procedure

First work the points along the governing vessel and small intestine meridians, holding each for three to five seconds. Next, stimulate the points shown on the large intestine, lung and bladder meridians. Finally, stimulate the points shown on the triple heater, pericardium and gall bladder meridians. Stimulate the meridian points from front to rear, top to bottom, doing each meridian line two times on both sides of your dog. Hold reactive points for ten to fifteen seconds.

Reactions to look for include front leg extension, neck twisting, muscle spasms, and avoidance.

Stretches

Do the deltoid/biceps stretch, shoulder extension, and shoulder rotation stretches. The shoulder will probably be restricted due to stiffness, so when you do the stretches, be careful to keep the stretch within your dog's comfort zone. As you proceed with treatments, the stretch of your dog should improve.

Frequency

Administer the acupressure treatment and stretches every other day for one week, or until the condition subsides. Do the acupressure treatment on one day and the stretches on the alternate day.

Important Points to be Worked

Meridian	Points	Meridian	Points
GV	12, 13 & 14	SI	3, 6, 7 & 8
LI	4, 10, 11 & 14	Lu	5 & 9
Bl	40 & 43	TH	4, 8, 10, 12 13 & 14
Pe	5 & 6	GB	21

SHOULDER SORENESS

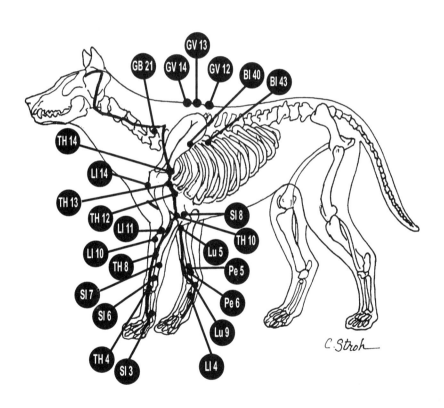

NOTE: See Chapter 3 For Location of Full Meridians

STIFLE PROBLEMS

Shows Up As • Lack of rear leg extension
             • Hind leg lameness
             • Subtle to moderate uneven rear leg stride
             • Crossing over or tracking wide

Refer to the drawing on the opposite page for the meridians and points to be worked.

Procedure

Stifle lameness can be rectified by working the stomach, bladder, spleen, gall bladder and kidney meridian points noted. Begin with points on the bladder meridian, working from the top to the bottom. Continue the same procedure for point work shown on the kidney, spleen, gall bladder and stomach meridians. Hold each point for three to five seconds. Stimulate the meridian points two times on both sides of your dog. Hold reactive points for ten to fifteen seconds.

Typical reactions include rear leg lifting, muscle spasms, avoidance and weight shifting.

Stretches

Perform the buttocks and stifle/pelvis extension stretches.

Frequency

Perform this acupressure treatment every other day for seven to ten days, or until the condition subsides. Perform stretches on the days between the acupressure treatment.

Important Points to be Worked

Meridian	Points	Meridian	Points
St	21, 25, 35, 38 & 41	Bl	20, 21 & 50
Sp	5 & 6	GB	30 & 34
Ki	8		

STIFLE PROBLEMS

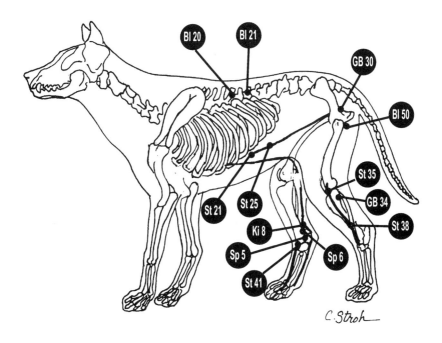

C. Stroh

NOTE: See Chapter 3 For Location of Full Meridians

LOWER BACK SORENESS

Shows Up As
- Stiff back movement
- Lack of loin flexibility
- Hind leg lameness
- Difficulty in getting up and/or lying down

Refer to the drawing on the opposite page for the meridians and points to be worked.

Procedure

This common canine ailment can be relieved by working points along the bladder, gall bladder, stomach, spleen, kidney, liver and conception vessel meridians. Begin with the bladder meridian, stimulating the points illustrated for three to five seconds. Repeat work on these points. Work the points on the gall bladder and stomach meridians two times, holding for three to five seconds. Finally, work the spleen, kidney, liver and conception vessel meridians, paying attention to the important points noted. Repeat the full treatment on the opposite side of your dog. Reactive points on any of the meridians should be held for ten to fifteen seconds or until a release of tension is felt. Complete the treatment by closing your dog twice on both sides of his body.

This ailment often produces reactions such as muscle spasms, rear leg extensions, tail crooking, excessive yawning and rear leg lifts.

Stretches

Perform all of the rear leg stretches and the neck stretch. Repeat stretches two times.

Frequency

Perform this acupressure treatment and these stretches every other day for ten days or until the condition subsides. Do the acupressure treatment one day and the stretches on the next.

Important Points to be Worked

Meridian	Points	Meridian	Points
Bl	20, 21, 23, 50 & 51	GB	29, 30 & 34
St	21, 25, 36, 38 & 41	Sp	5 & 6
Ki	7 & 8	Liv	8
CV	6 (See page 50 for location)		

LOWER BACK SORNESS

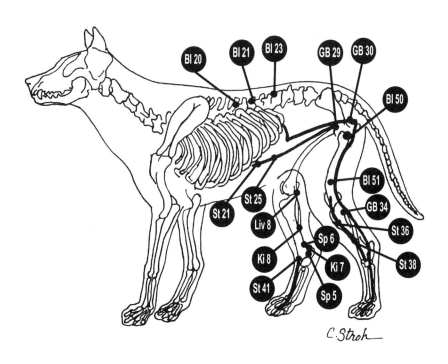

NOTE: See Chapter 3 For Location of Full Meridians

HIP PROBLEMS

Shows Up As
- Hind leg lameness
- Difficulty lying down and/or standing up
- Inability to extend or retract hind leg

Refer to the drawing on the opposite page for the meridians and points to be worked.

Procedure

Hip soreness can be relieved by stimulating the points shown on the opposite page. Open your dog as described in Chapter 6. Stimulate the bladder meridian beginning at the shoulders and running its entire length. Pay particular attention to bladder points 20, 21 and 50 as these may well be sensitive to stimulation and/or produce reactions. Hold the points for three to eight seconds, working front to back. Next work the gall bladder meridian with point work concentrated at points 29 and 30. Then work the stomach meridian from the stifle through its termination point at the foot, paying attention to points 21 and 25. Finally, work the spleen and kidney meridians. Hold points which show a reaction for 10 to 15 seconds. Complete with the closing of your choice.

Typical reactions will include moving the body away from or into point stimulation, licking and salivation, deep sighs, yawning or hind leg stretching.

Stretches

Do the buttocks, stifle/pelvis and hip flexion stretches. However, if soreness is too pronounced, do just the acupressure treatment until soreness subsides and then perform the stretches.

Frequency

Perform this acupressure treatment every other day for eight to twelve days, or until the condition subsides. Perform stretches on the days between the acupressure treatment.

Important Points to be Worked

Meridian	Points	Meridian	Points
Bl	20, 21, 50, 54 & 60	St	21, 25 & 36
GB	29, 30, & 39	Sp	6
Ki	8	Liv	2 & 8
GV	4		

HIP PROBLEMS

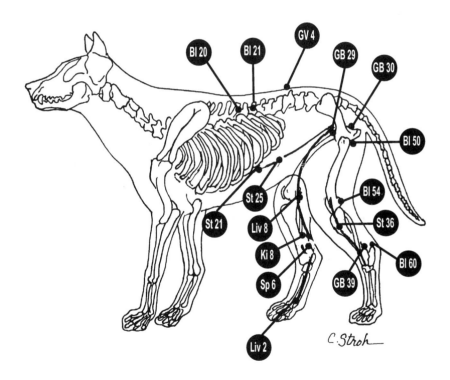

NOTE: See Chapter 3 For Location of Full Meridians

POINTS FOR CALMING YOUR DOG

Shows Up As
- Aggressiveness
- Hyperactivity
- Limited attention span

Refer to the drawing on the opposite page for the meridians and points to be worked.

Procedure/Use

In addition to a complete acupressure treatment, we have found the points noted on the opposite page to be helpful in calming and relieving tension in a variety of animals. The points may be used in succession, beginning with the governing vessel Yin-Tang point, or "randomly" as your dog will allow if he is in an agitated state.

Frequency

Stimulate points until the dog shows a state of release or relaxation. Depending on the situation, it may take from several minutes to one half hour to achieve a relaxed and quiet state. As you work these points more frequently on your dog, the response time leading to relaxation will become shorter.

Important Points to be Worked

Meridian	Points	Meridian	Points
GV	Yin-Tang	CV	12, 14 & 17
Ht	6 & 7	Liv	2 & 3
Bl	15 & 18		

POINTS FOR CALMING YOUR DOG

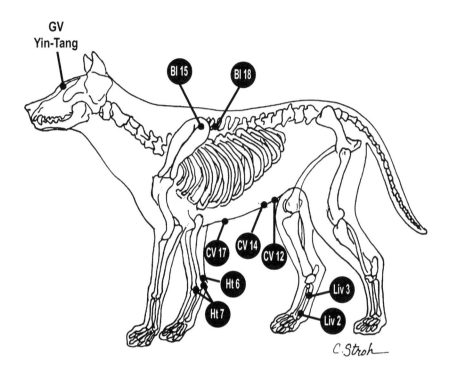

NOTE: See Chapter 3 For Location of Full Meridians

10. BIBLIOGRAPHY

Altman, Sheldon, DVM. *An Introduction to Acupuncture for Animals*. Chen's Corporation, Monterey Park, CA. 1981.

Becker, Robert, O. & Selden, Gary. *The Body Electric*. Quill, New York, NY. 1985.

Beinfield, Harriet, L.Ac. & Korngold, Efrem, L. Ac., OMD. *Between Heaven and Earth, A Guide to Chinese Medicine*. Ballentine Books, New York, NY. 1991.

Connelly, Dianne, M., Ph.D., M. Ac. *Traditional Acupuncture: The Law of the Five Elements*. The Centre for Traditional Acupuncture, Columbia, MD. 1989.

Fox, Michael W. Ph.D., D.Sc. *The Healing Touch*. New Market Press, New York, NY. 1990.

Gerber, Richard, MD. *Vibrational Medicine*. Bear & Co., Santa Fe, N M. 1988 .

Jarmey, Chris & Tindall, John. *Acupressure for Common Ailments*. Simon & Schuster Inc., New York, NY. 1991.

Kaptchuk, Ted, OMD. *The Web That Has No Weaver, Understanding Chinese Medicine*. Congdon & Weed, Inc., New York, NY. 1983.

International Veterinary Acupuncture Society, The. *Chinese Acupuncture, 5,000 Year Old Oriental Art of Healing*.

Masunaga, Shizuto & Ohashi, Wataru. Zen Shiatsu, *How to Harmonize Yin & Yang for Better Health*. Japan Publications Inc., Tokyo & New York. 1977.

Namokoshi, Tory. *The Complete Book of Shiatsu Therapy*. Japan Publications, Inc., New York & Tokyo. 1981.

Serizawa, Katsusuke. *Tsubo Vital Points for Oriental Therapy.* Japan Publications Inc., Tokyo & New York. 1976.

Schoen, Allen, M. *Veterinary Acupuncture, Ancient Art to Modern Medicine.* American Veterinary Publications, Inc., Goleta, CA. 1994.

Sohn, Tina. Amma, *The Ancient Art of Oriental Healing.* Healing Arts Press, Rochester, Vermont. 1988.

Mann, Felix, MD. Acupuncture, *The Ancient Chinese Art of Healing and How It Works Scientifically.* Vintage Books, New York, NY. 1973.

Stein, Diane. *Natural Healing for Dogs and Cats.* The Crossing Press, Freedom, CA. 1993.

Louise Wensenl, MD. *Acupressure for Americans.* Reston Publishing Co, Inc., Reston, VA. 1980.

Stux, Gabriel, & Pomeranz, Bruce. *Basics of Acupuncture.* Springer-Verlag, Berlin, Heidelberg, New York. 1991.

Zidonis, Nancy A., & Soderberg, Marie K. *Equine Acupressure, A Treatment Workbook.* Equine Acupressure, Inc., Parker, CO. 1992.

CANINE ACUPRESSURE

Please send me_____ copy/copies of **Canine Acupressure, A Treatment Workbook** @ $18.00 plus $.63 tax per copy, Colorado residents only.

Shipping and Handling

1-5 books $3.00 per book

5-10 books $2.50 per book

Books _____

Tax _____

Shipping/Handling _____

TOTAL FOR ORDER _____

Payment and Shipping Information

Name: _____

Address:_____

City/State: _____

Zip Code:_____

Phone: _____

Form of Payment

____Check _____Money Order _____MasterCard ____VISA

MC/VISA Account # _____

Expiration date: _____

Signature: _____

Please mail order form with payment to:
Equine Acupressure, Inc.
P.O. Box 123 • Parker, CO 80134
or call in your order to 303-841-7211
303-841-6939 Fax

CLINICS AND SEMINARS AVAILABLE
CALL FOR INFORMATION
